FIRST AID at work

A text for all HSE Approved and Recognised courses and a reference in particular, for qualified First Aiders

Author: Seb Sevett

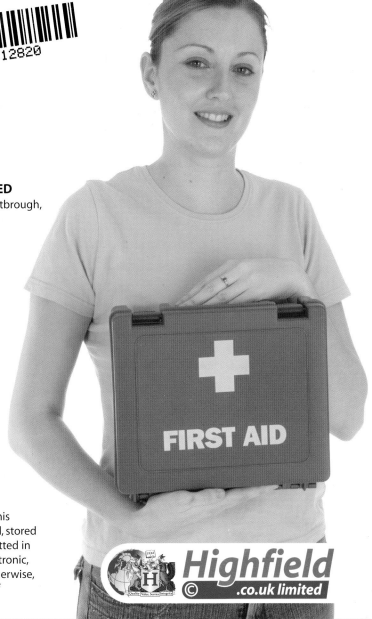

D1312820

PUBLISHED BY
© **HIGHFIELD.CO.UK LIMITED**
"Vue Pointe", Spinney Hill, Sprotbrough,
Doncaster, DN5 7LY, UK
Tel: +44 0845 2260350
Fax: +44 0845 2260360
E-mail: Richard@highfield.co.uk

Websites:
www.highfield.co.uk
www.highfield.co.uk/firstaid

ISBN 1 904 544 66 5

THIRD EDITION
May 2006

First edition - February 2006
Second edition - April 2006

FIRST AID

At some point in your life you may be faced with a situation where emergency aid is required. This may be at home, at work or in the street.

The question you have to ask yourself is:

Will I know what to do if the situation arises?

Attending a First Aid course is the first step in gaining the necessary knowledge and skills. Keeping this book handy at work or at home will help to keep that knowledge refreshed and you prepared if that unfortunate situation should arise.

This book is intended primarily as a source of reference on your First Aid course and sets out the recommended procedures currently adopted for First Aid in the United Kingdom. The information is correct at the time of publication and is in accordance with The European Resuscitation Council Guidelines 2005 and other professional bodies involved in emergency care.

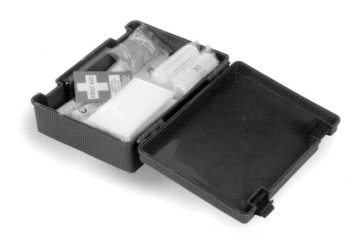

WELCOME

This book provides step-by-step, easy to understand procedures for dealing with everyday emergencies that occur at work or at home. It is designed to play an integral part of your First Aid course.

Each section closely follows the sessions that your instructor will teach with a full description of the background, recognition features and treatment of a particular illness or injury.

This book is not intended to replace the need for professional medical care but to provide that vital information needed in those first few minutes when dealing with sudden injury or illness.

WELCOME TO YOUR FIRST AID COURSE

Delegate name:

Olivia Moore

Course start date:

Course end date:

Course Instructor:

Additional details (if any):

FIRST AID at work

Contents

CONTENTS

CONTENTS   Page

FIRST AID at work

Contents

CONTENTS   Page

CONTENTS   Page

CONTENTS   Page

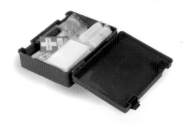

THE FIRST AIDER

The term First Aider generally applies to someone who has attended a First Aid At Work course and has successfully passed the final assessment necessary to gain the qualification. To become a First Aider in the workplace you will need to attend and successfully complete the assessment of a Health & Safety Executive approved First Aid course. This qualification is valid for a period of three years. In order to remain qualified you must undergo re-qualification by attending a 2-day refresher course before your qualification lapses.

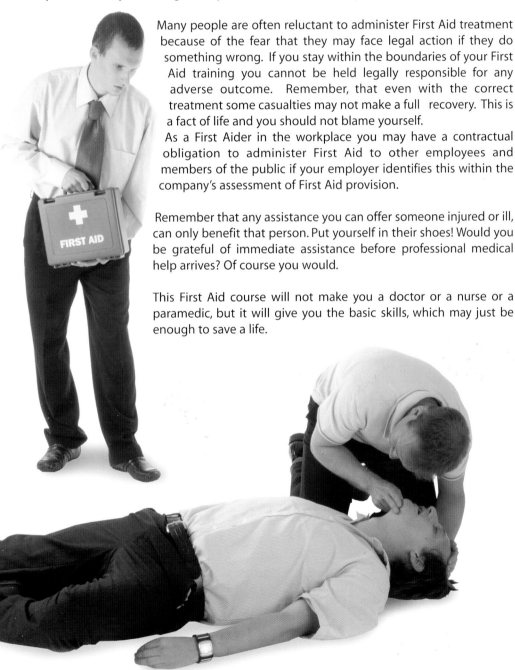

Many people are often reluctant to administer First Aid treatment because of the fear that they may face legal action if they do something wrong. If you stay within the boundaries of your First Aid training you cannot be held legally responsible for any adverse outcome. Remember, that even with the correct treatment some casualties may not make a full recovery. This is a fact of life and you should not blame yourself.

As a First Aider in the workplace you may have a contractual obligation to administer First Aid to other employees and members of the public if your employer identifies this within the company's assessment of First Aid provision.

Remember that any assistance you can offer someone injured or ill, can only benefit that person. Put yourself in their shoes! Would you be grateful of immediate assistance before professional medical help arrives? Of course you would.

This First Aid course will not make you a doctor or a nurse or a paramedic, but it will give you the basic skills, which may just be enough to save a life.

FIRST AID at work

DEFINITION OF FIRST AID

First Aid is the initial or immediate assistance given to someone who has been injured or taken ill before the arrival of qualified medical assistance.

THE AIMS OF FIRST AID

TO PRESERVE LIFE
Always check for safety to you, the casualty and any bystanders. Carry out the necessary checks for maintaining the airway, breathing and circulation and be prepared to carry out lifesaving emergency First Aid.

PREVENT THE CONDITION FROM WORSENING
Assess the casualty's injuries or illness by carrying out a thorough examination. Prioritize and treat life-threatening conditions first. Do not move casualties unless absolutely necessary.

PROMOTE RECOVERY
Only give First Aid treatment in accordance with your training. Provide care with confidence and try to relieve any discomfort and anxiety. Reassure the casualty and arrange for any emergency medical care.

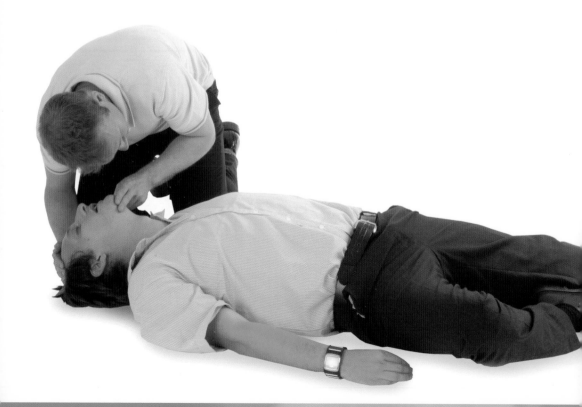

FIRST AID IN THE WORKPLACE

Anyone may give First Aid treatment to the sick or injured in the home or on the street. This may be due to the fact that they are trained or because they are the first person on the scene. First Aid within the workplace is governed by legislation.

As a First Aider in the workplace it is important to have an understanding of how various Acts and Regulations affect the provision of First Aid and the responsibilities placed upon your employer and yourself.

HEALTH & SAFETY ACTS AND REGULATIONS

THE HEALTH AND SAFETY AT WORK ACT 1974
Requires employers to ensure, so far as is reasonably practicable, the health, safety and welfare at work of all their employees. This also extends to non-employees such as outside contractors and members of the public.

THE MANAGEMENT OF THE HEALTH AND SAFETY AT WORK REGULATIONS 1999
Requires employers to make a suitable and sufficient assessment of the risks to health and safety of all their employees. Information gathered from this risk assessment can help the employer to carry out the assessment for First Aid needs.

THE HEALTH AND SAFETY (FIRST AID) REGULATIONS 1981
Employers are required to provide adequate personnel, training, equipment and facilities to render First Aid to their employees should they become injured or taken ill at work.

FIRST AID AT WORK PROVISION

As a First Aider you should liaise with your company's management and other First Aiders:

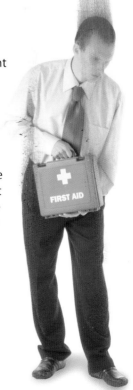

○ To ensure that the provision of First Aid is organised
○ To ensure adequate First Aid kits are available
○ To keep records and reports

Where the First Aid assessment identifies a need for people to be available for rendering First Aid, the employer should ensure that they are provided in sufficient numbers and at appropriate locations to enable First Aid to be administered without delay should the occasion arise.

Guidance on the appropriate numbers of First Aiders in a particular workplace is set out in the Health & Safety (First Aid) Regulations 1981, Approved Code of Practice (ACOP) and Guidance publication. This also contains guidance on the content and quantity of First Aid containers.

Section 3

FIRST AID CONTAINERS AND THEIR CONTENTS

First Aid containers:
- ○ Keep clean and free from dust
- ○ Protect contents from damp
- ○ If possible make accessible, preferably locate near to hand washing facilities
- ○ Should be green with a white cross
- ○ Examine regularly and restock after use
- ○ Discard out-of-date items
- ○ Keep a sufficient supply

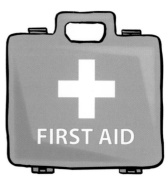

FIRST AID

The contents of a First Aid container will be determined from the information gathered in the company assessment of First Aid needs. For example, the risk assessment of a building site would determine a higher risk factor than that of a small office. Therefore, the quantity of First Aid materials would be greater.

There is no mandatory list of materials that should be kept in a First Aid container but the Approved Code of Practice gives guidance on the minimum content that should be made available where no special risks are involved.

MINIMUM SUGGESTED CONTENTS:
- ○ A guidance leaflet
- ○ 20 adhesive dressings
  (individually wrapped and assorted sizes)
- ○ 2 sterile eye pads
- ○ 6 triangular bandages
  (individually wrapped and sterile)
- ○ 6 medium sterile wound dressings
  (individually wrapped and un-medicated)
- ○ 2 large sterile wound dressings
  (individually wrapped and un-medicated)
- ○ 6 safety pins
- ○ Disposable gloves

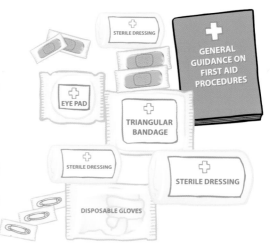

Should the assessment conclude the need for such items, employers may include additional materials within the container or kept separate in a First Aid room:
- ○ Blunt tipped scissors
- ○ Non-alcoholic wipes
- ○ Micropore tape
- ○ Disposable apron
- ○ Protective equipment
- ○ Clinical waste bag
- ○ Special burns dressings

No creams, lotions, potions, medicines or tablets are permitted

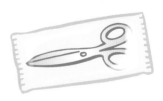

EYE IRRIGATION

Where no fresh mains tap water is available, a litre of sterile eyewash should be made available for the purpose of eye irrigation.

Do not use if the seal on the container is broken and never re-use once it has been opened. Discard any remaining contents along with the container.

ACCIDENT AND INCIDENT REPORTING

Following any accident or incident it is important to record all details relating to the situation.

1. **PERSON AFFECTED/INJURED**

Name ....

Home address ....

....

Occupation .... Works number ....

2. **PERSON REPORTING THE INCIDENT**

Name ....

Home address ....

....

Occupation ....

Department .... Date ..../........../..........

3. **ABOUT THE ACCIDENT/INCIDENT**

Date ..../........../.......... Time ....

Place ....

Equipment/machinery involved ....

....

4. **DESCRIPTION OF THE INCIDENT**

Cause ....

....

Nature ....

....

Treatment given ....

....

Material used ....

Signed .... Date ..../......./......

Reportable under RIDDOR (if appropriate)   YES   NO

The information contained in the accident book can often help employers to identify accident trends and improve the general Health & Safety of the workplace. These records may also be required for insurance and investigative purposes. In 2003 a new accident book was introduced to comply with data protection legislation. It is designed so that any individual recording an accident is unable to access personal details of previous records.

Section 3

REPORTING OF INJURIES, DISEASES AND DANGEROUS OCCURRENCES REGULATIONS (RIDDOR) *(legal requirement)*

For serious accidents/incidents at work the employer is required to notify their local authority, the HSE or the incident contact centre in Caerphilly (UK).

The First Aider may not be directly responsible for completing the RIDDOR report, but should ensure that management or the Health & Safety Officer receives the correct information contained within the accident book.

ACCIDENTS AND INCIDENTS THAT REQUIRE IMMEDIATE REPORTING
○ Deaths
○ Major injuries - such as amputations, loss of sight and most fractures.

OVER THREE DAY INJURIES
Employers must notify within 10 days any injury that causes an employee to be off work or not able to perform their usual job for more than three days. These are reported on an F2508 form.

Work-related ill health should be notified within 10 days of diagnosis on an F2508a form.

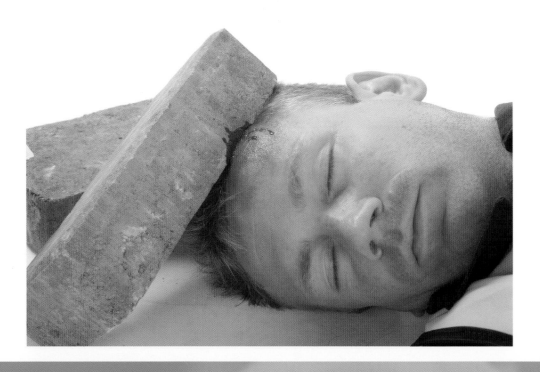

RESPONSIBILITIES OF THE FIRST AIDER

In any situation where the assistance of a First Aider is required, the First Aider should follow an organized assessment of both the surroundings and the casualty or casualties.

ARRIVAL AT THE SCENE
- Assess the situation
- Make the area safe if possible
- Ask questions about the situation
- Obtain help from others
- Send for help

Always ensure that it is safe for you to approach a casualty before attempting to carry out any treatment. Your safety comes first, so do not put yourself in any danger. Ask what happened, if anyone saw the incident or if there are any other trained personnel available. Do not allow yourself to become isolated when dealing with emergency situations. Take control and obtain assistance from those around you, as their help may be required with the casualty or in sending them for a First Aid box and calling the Emergency Services. You may be dealing with multiple casualties, so assistance is vital.

DEALING WITH CASUALTIES
- Protect yourself
- Check for unconsciousness
- Ensure the airway is open and your casualty is breathing
- Assess the extent of the injury or illness
- Treat in order of priority
- Be calm and confident
- Make sure that qualified help has been called for as soon as you have determined the extent of the injury or illness

CONTACTING THE EMERGENCY SERVICES

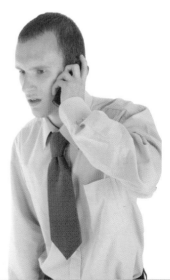

MAKING THE PHONE CALL
- State which service you require
- Give your telephone number
- State your exact location
- State type of incident
- Give number of casualties
- State type and extent of the injuries
- State dangerous hazards

The European Union Emergency number 112 is now in operation as well as 999.

PRIORITIES OF FIRST AID TREATMENT

Wear gloves to protect both yourself and the casualty. This will help to prevent the risk of cross-infection. Carry out a primary survey and quickly assess the condition of the casualty. Deal with life-threatening conditions first.
Treat in the correct order:

○ Breathing
○ Bleeding
○ Bones
○ Other conditions (treat and prioritise accordingly)

THE CLEARING UP PROCESS

Give an accurate account of the situation to the Emergency Services. Complete the accident book and RIDDOR form if necessary. Wear protective clothing and clean up any blood or bodily fluids. Dispose of any contaminated materials in a yellow biohazard bag for incineration. You may need to talk about the incident, especially if the treatment was unsuccessful and you feel that you are unable to cope with your feelings.

CASUALTY COMMUNICATION

Someone who is sick or injured will be scared and may not understand what is being said or done. Therefore, gestures, body language and attitude towards the casualty are critically important in gaining their trust.

MAKE AND KEEP EYE CONTACT WITH YOUR CASUALTY AT ALL TIMES

Give your casualty your undivided attention. This will let the casualty know that he or she is your top priority. Look the casualty in the eye to establish rapport. Establishing rapport is building a trusting relationship with your casualty.

TELL YOUR CASUALTY THE TRUTH

Even if you have something to say that is very unpleasant, telling the truth is better than lying. Lying will destroy the casualty's trust in you and decreases your confidence.

USE LANGUAGE THAT THE CASUALTY CAN UNDERSTAND

Do not talk up or down to the casualty in any way. Avoid technical medical terms that the casualty may not understand.

BE CAREFUL OF WHAT YOU SAY ABOUT THE CASUALTY TO OTHERS

A casualty may only hear part of what is said. As a result, the casualty may seriously misinterpret what was said. Assume that the casualty can hear every word you say even if the casualty appears to be unconscious.

BE AWARE OF YOUR BODY LANGUAGE

Non-verbal communication is extremely important when dealing with casualties. In stressful situations casualties may misinterpret your movements and gestures. Be particularly careful not to appear threatening. Position yourself on a level with the casualty when it is practical to do so.

ALWAYS SPEAK SLOWLY, CLEARLY AND DISTINCTLY
Use the casualty's proper name if you know it. Ask the casualty what they would like to be called.

IF THE CASUALTY'S HEARING IS IMPAIRED, SPEAK CLEARLY AND FACE THEM IN ORDER FOR THEM TO READ YOUR LIPS
Do not shout. Shouting will not make it easier for the casualty to understand you. Never use baby talk with elderly casualties.

ALLOW TIME FOR THE CASUALTY TO ANSWER OR RESPOND TO YOUR QUESTIONS
Sick or injured people may need time to answer even simple questions.

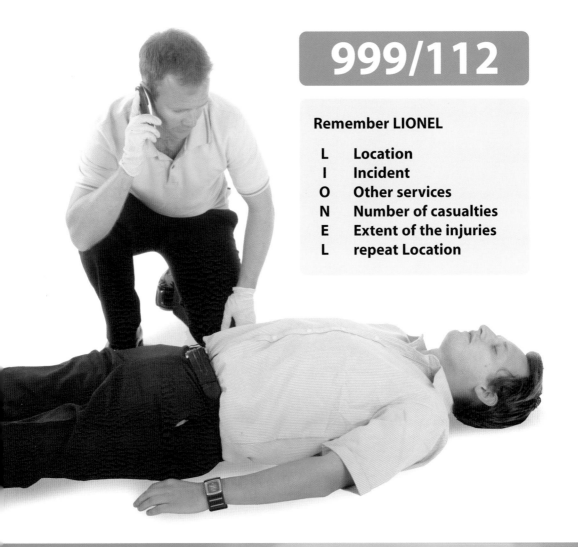

999/112

Remember LIONEL

L	Location
I	Incident
O	Other services
N	Number of casualties
E	Extent of the injuries
L	repeat Location

Section 5

FACTORS INVOLVED IN AN EMERGENCY

When alerted to a possible emergency, the first thing to consider is an assessment of the area for any dangers to you, the casualty and any bystanders.

In assessing the area before approaching the casualty, you should follow an action plan.

STOP   Take a deep breath and have a good look around you

ENVIRONMENT   Consider your limitations. Are you confident and able to cope when dealing with a collapsed building or someone who is drowning?

TRAFFIC   Remain alert. Ask for assistance in stopping approaching vehicles. All engines should be turned off.

UNKNOWN   Hazards such as gas, electricity, chemicals

PROTECT   Use protective clothing or equipment to prevent cross-infection or contamination

POSSIBLE HAZARDS
Hazards may include:
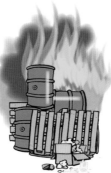
- Traffic
- Electricity
- Water
- Buildings
- Fire
- Chemicals
- Smoke and gas
- Bystanders

ROAD TRAFFIC ACCIDENTS

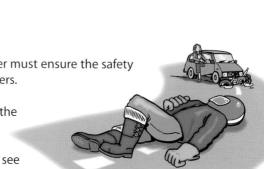

Whatever the circumstances, the First Aider must ensure the safety of themselves, any casualties and bystanders.

This may involve obtaining help to make the area safe before approaching any casualties. Ask any bystanders to park their vehicles where oncoming traffic can see their hazard lights flashing.

ON REACHING A VEHICLE AT AN EMERGENCY THE FIRST AIDER SHOULD:
- Check that the ignition key is turned off
- Put the vehicle in neutral with the handbrake on
- **Not** allow bystanders to smoke in case there is leaking fuel
- Ensure that the Emergency Services are called
- **Not** move injured casualties unless absolutely necessary

○ Follow the procedures for a primary assessment (Section 6)
○ Be aware of possible spinal injury
○ Be prepared to resuscitate
○ If a casualty is unconscious but breathing, place them in the recovery position
○ Treat any bleeding and check for other injuries

When a casualty is severely injured and still seated in a vehicle, it is advisable not to cause any movement unless their airway and breathing is impaired.

If the accident involves motorcycles, riders may have multiple injuries and possible spinal damage, so extra care should be taken if you have to remove a crash helmet.

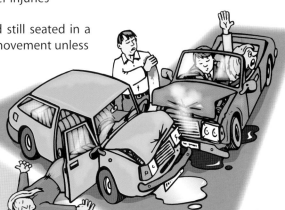

Remove the visor and carry out your primary assessment (Section 6).

If the casualty is breathing with no apparent blockage of the airway leave the helmet in place.

If the casualty is not breathing and you cannot resuscitate through the visor opening you will have to remove the helmet. Two people should do this. One person to stabilize the head and neck and the other to remove the strap and pull the helmet out sideways to loosen the grip around the ears. By lifting the helmet up to clear the chin, you should now be able to tilt it forwards from the back of the skull. *AVOID ANY MOVEMENT OF THE HEAD AND NECK*

ELECTRICITY – DOMESTIC

Although the domestic electricity supply is low voltage, contact with a live conductor can cause serious injury or death.

Make the area safe by breaking the electrical contact in the easiest but safest manner. If it is possible to remove an appliance plug from the power supply point do so, as this will stop the flow of electricity. You should not rely purely on switching off the power at the switch because it is possible for electricity to flow even after this has been turned off. Alternatively, the power should be turned off from the mains supply to ensure complete safety for all concerned.

When it is safe to proceed, assess the casualty's airway and breathing and be prepared to resuscitate.

The First Aider should then check for any burns. Look carefully for an exit burn as this is likely to be the most serious secondary injury.

ELECTRICITY – HIGH VOLTAGE

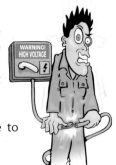

In emergencies involving overhead power cables or the high voltage supply that can be found in large factories, immediately call the Emergency Services to ensure that the Power Company shuts down the power supply. Make sure that you and any bystander remain at least 18 metres from the cables or supply.

Advise any people who may be trapped in a vehicle or structure to remain where they are and to avoid any contact with metal.

STRUCTURAL DAMAGE

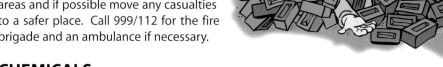

On building sites or when a building is collapsing due to structural damage, there may be the danger of falling debris or collapsing floors. Keep all bystanders away from the areas and if possible move any casualties to a safer place. Call 999/112 for the fire brigade and an ambulance if necessary.

CHEMICALS

When chemical spills occur within the workplace, the First Aider should follow the guidelines that have been put in place following the COSHH assessment and allow trained personnel to deal with the spillage.

The First Aider may have to treat casualties for chemical burns and extreme care should be taken to avoid contamination.

Wear protective clothing and do not attempt to use any specific neutralizing agents unless trained to do so.

Use running water for a minimum of 20 minutes if applicable.

Chemical burns are covered in greater detail in Section 16.

WATER

In deep or fast-flowing water, any form of rescue can be extremely dangerous. Unless you have been properly trained to perform such a rescue, it is advisable to stay out of the water and to use an indirect method of rescue.

If the casualty is conscious use a rope, a pole or an item of clothing for the casualty to grasp. If they are further away, try throwing some form of floatation device such as a plastic container.

Casualties who have fallen or jumped into shallow water may have injured their spine. Care should be taken to avoid further damage (Section 17).

The casualty may become extremely cold due to prolonged exposure that could lead to hypothermia. Try to keep them warm and avoid movement (Section 19).

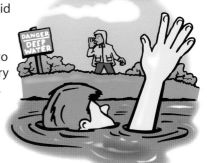

Any person who has been rescued from water should receive medical attention.

FIRE

When fire is present at an emergency, the First Aider must be aware of the serious risk to life when entering a burning building or room. Fire produces toxic fumes as well as the danger from heat and smoke.

If caught in a smoke-filled area, the First Aider should drop to the floor and attempt to crawl to safety.

Treatment for casualties with smoke inhalation injuries is covered in Section 10.

SECTION SUMMARY

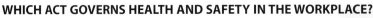

THE MAIN AIMS OF FIRST AID:
- Preserve life
- Prevent the condition from worsening
- Promote recovery

WHICH ACT GOVERNS HEALTH AND SAFETY IN THE WORKPLACE?
- The Health & Safety at Work Act 1974

WHICH REGULATION GOVERNS FIRST AID IN THE WORKPLACE?
- The Health & Safety First Aid Regulations 1981

THE SUGGESTED CONTENTS OF A BASIC FIRST AID KIT:
- Guidance card
- 20 Adhesive dressings
- 2 Sterile eye pads
- 6 Medium sterile dressings
- 2 Large sterile dressings
- 6 Safety pins
- 6 Triangular bandages
- Disposable gloves

AS A FIRST AIDER YOU SHOULD LIAISE WITH MANAGEMENT AND OTHER FIRST AIDERS:
- To ensure that the provision of First Aid is organized
- To ensure that adequate First Aid kits are available
- To keep records and reports

WHEN APPROACHING AN INCIDENT YOU SHOULD CONSIDER:
- Safety of yourself, the casualty and any bystanders
- Are you able to deal with the situation?
- Is there any help available?
- How many casualties are there?
- Are there any unknown hazards such as gas or chemicals?

PRIORITISE THE INJURIES WHEN DEALING WITH YOUR CASUALTY
- Breathing
- Bleeding
- Bones
- Other conditions (treat and prioritise accordingly)

AFTER DEALING WITH ANY INCIDENT YOU SHOULD:
- Clean up any blood, vomit and soiled dressings and use the correct disposal procedure
- Restock the First Aid kit
- Complete the accident report book
- Report the incident to your manager
- Ensure that the area is safe before allowing any access

PRIMARY ASSESSMENT

Having assessed the surrounding area for any dangers and ensured that it is safe to approach the casualty you should now carry out a primary assessment of the casualty to identify any life-threatening conditions.

You should remember that life-threatening conditions that need emergency aid must take priority over any other First Aid treatment.

APPROACHING THE CASUALTY
○ Approach the casualty from their side or their feet
○ Talk to the casualty as you approach to see if they are alert
○ Kneel down by their side

CHECKING FOR A RESPONSE
○ Give a verbal command into both ears e.g. open your eyes, talk to me
○ Speak loudly and calmly
○ Gently shake the shoulders

If the casualty is responsive but has suffered severe injuries leave them in the position found and treat accordingly. Otherwise establish the possible cause of the collapse. Treat any injuries and obtain medical assistance if necessary.

If the casualty does not respond shout for help to attract the attention of others.

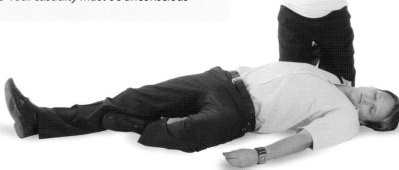

Remember the acronym

A	Alert	*Is your casualty completely responsive?*
V	Voice	*Does your casualty respond to a voice command?*
P	Pain	*Does your casualty respond to pain only?*
U	Unresponsive	*Your casualty must be unconscious*

OPENING THE AIRWAY

If the casualty does not respond, the airway needs protecting. If necessary turn the unconscious casualty into the face-up position.

The airway must be open to do this we use the head-tilt-chin-lift manoeuvre.

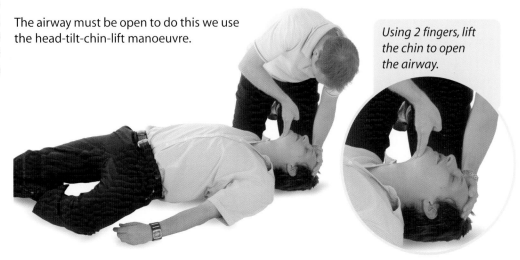

Using 2 fingers, lift the chin to open the airway.

With one hand on the casualty's forehead tilt back the head and using 2 fingers of your other hand, lift the chin to fully open the airway.

The tongue is attached to the lower jaw and this action prevents the tongue from falling back and blocking the airway.

Lift the chin without tilting the head.

CHECKING FOR NORMAL BREATHING

With the airway open and maintained, check for normal breathing.

Do this for up to ten seconds by:
LOOK:
For movement of the chest and upper abdomen
LISTEN:
For breathing by placing one ear above the casualty's mouth and nose
FEEL:
For breath on your cheek as it escapes from the mouth or nose

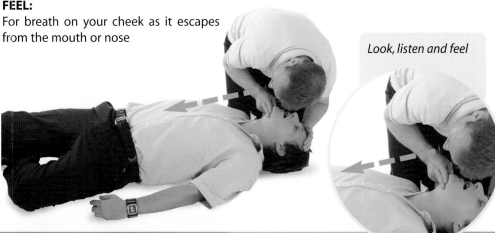

Look, listen and feel

IS THE CASUALTY BREATHING NORMALLY?
If the casualty is unconscious and breathing normally check for any injuries and treat accordingly. Place in the recovery position (Section 7).

If the casualty is not breathing normally, send a bystander to call 999/112 for an ambulance.

If you are on your own you must go yourself as soon as you have established your casualty is not breathing normally. Upon your return, start chest compressions immediately (Section 9).

PRIMARY ASSESSMENT

D Danger	Make sure the area is safe before you approach	
R Response	Check to see if the casualty responds to verbal commands or a pain stimulus	
	SHOUT FOR HELP	
A Airway	Open the airway by tilting the head back and lifting the chin with two fingers	
B Breathing	Look, listen and feel for normal breathing for up to ten seconds	

AGONAL GASPS
There will be reference throughout this manual to your casualty breathing normally.

It is important to understand that in up to 40% of Cardiac Arrest victims, Agonal Gasps are present. This would indicate that your casualty is not breathing normally.

Agonal Gasping is best described as infrequent, irregular breathing.

You must start CPR if your casualty is unconscious and not breathing normally.

It must be emphasised that Agonal Gasps occur commonly in the first few minutes after sudden Cardiac Arrest. They are an indication for starting CPR immediately and should not be confused with normal breathing.

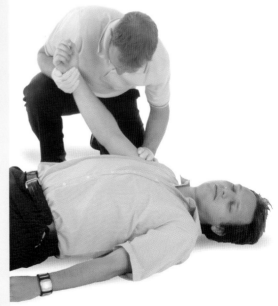

*Once you have completed **D.R.A.B.** prepare to move on to your secondary assessment of the casualty*

SECONDARY ASSESSMENT

Once you have completed your primary assessment and made sure that the casualty is out of immediate danger, you will need to make an assessment of the casualty's injuries and condition.

The way in which you carry out the steps will depend on whether the casualty is alert and responsive or unconscious.

ASSESSMENT OF THE CASUALTY'S CONDITION
The three key factors involved in assessing a casualty's condition are:

HISTORY
○ Can the casualty tell you what happened and explain any medical history?
○ Did anyone see what happened?
○ Look at the surroundings as this may give you a clue e.g. fallen from a ladder
○ Is there evidence of substance abuse?
○ Is the casualty wearing a medical warning bracelet or pendant?
○ The age and general condition of the casualty may affect the extent of any injuries
○ Find out their name and any other details

SIGNS
These are what you can see, feel, smell and hear. Some signs may be evident but others may only be found by carrying out a complete examination of the casualty.

SYMPTOMS
These are what the casualty feels. The casualty may feel nauseous, suffering with pain, feeling weak and may have a headache. Encourage them to explain. Be patient and listen to the casualty.

Having found out the history of the casualty and the incident, you can move to the next phase of the secondary assessment where you are carefully looking and feeling for any signs of injury or any other indication of the casualty's condition.

During the assessment it is very important to talk to the casualty even if they are unconscious. Always explain what you are doing and constantly evaluate the casualty's level of consciousness and breathing.

Protect yourself and the casualty by wearing disposable gloves.

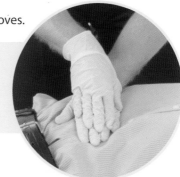

Remember to wear disposable gloves when working with a casualty.

THE TOP-TO-TOE SURVEY

1 HEAD AND FACE

First, make sure the nose and mouth are clear and the casualty is breathing normally. Carefully look at the face, scalp, ears, eyes, nose and mouth for any bleeding, bumps, swelling or depression. Remove spectacles. Examine eyes for unequal pupils. Look for any fluid drainage from ears and nose. Smell the casualty's breath for alcohol or unusual odour. Note the colour, temperature and state of the skin and lips.

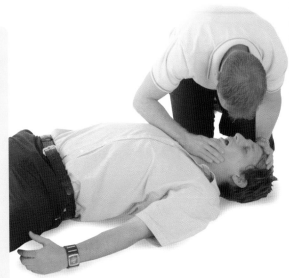

2 NECK

Loosen clothing around the neck and look for any medical advice medallions. Check carotid pulse for the benefit of monitoring only. Look at the head, neck and cervical spine for any obvious injuries or swelling. Gently feel the cervical spine for deformity or tenderness. Ask a responsive casualty if they feel any pain or tenderness.

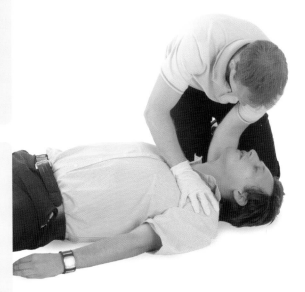

3 CHEST AND SHOULDERS

Look for any signs of injury. Gently press on the ribs to determine if there is any tenderness. Do not press on bruises or breaks in the skin. Look for the normal rise and fall of the chest with the breathing process. Gently feel along the collarbones and the shoulders for any deformity, irregularity or tenderness.

4 ARMS

Look for bruising, swelling, obvious deformities and bleeding. Feel along the arms for tenderness and pain. Look for needle marks and medical bracelets. Monitor the radial pulse.

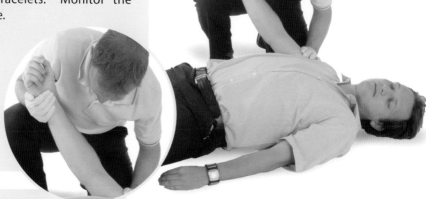

Check the arms.
Look for needle traces.

5 SPINE

Check as much of the spine as possible. Do not move the casualty. Check for tenderness, deformity and loss of sensation.

6 PELVIS

Feel both sides of the hips and gently squeeze the pelvis looking for signs of fracture or deformity.

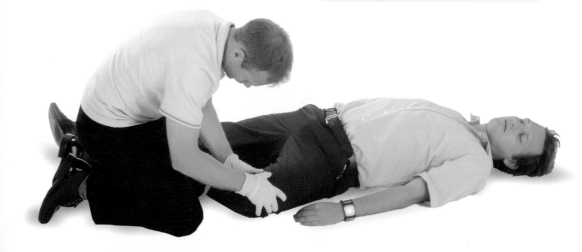

7 ABDOMEN

Look first for any signs of obvious injury including swelling and bruising. Ask if there is any pain or tenderness as you press over the abdomen and note any rigidity.

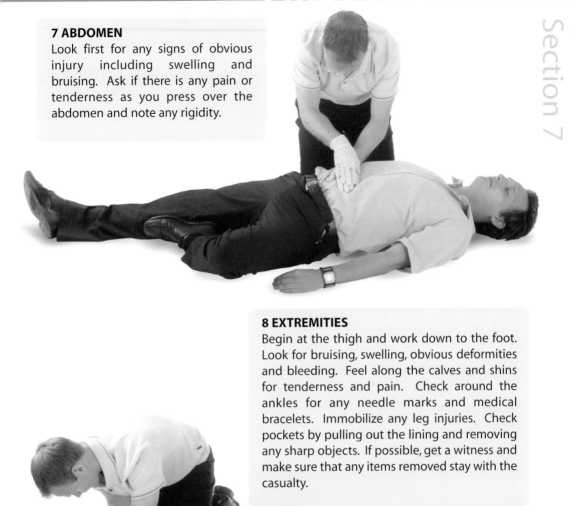

8 EXTREMITIES

Begin at the thigh and work down to the foot. Look for bruising, swelling, obvious deformities and bleeding. Feel along the calves and shins for tenderness and pain. Check around the ankles for any needle marks and medical bracelets. Immobilize any leg injuries. Check pockets by pulling out the lining and removing any sharp objects. If possible, get a witness and make sure that any items removed stay with the casualty.

A top-to-toe survey should be thorough, complete and carried out on all casualties when you suspect injury or when you are unsure of the circumstances leading to the incident.

Some casualties may be found lying on their front or in an awkward position so when you have established that the casualty is out of immediate danger i.e. breathing and no major bleeding, you should examine the casualty in the position found.

Only turn a breathing casualty from their front onto their back if you are unable to carry out a thorough survey or control any major bleeding.

Section 7

MANAGEMENT OF THE UNCONSCIOUS CASUALTY

THE RECOVERY POSITION

The recovery position is used to maintain a clear airway and assist spontaneous breathing. It also helps excretions such as vomit to drain from the mouth when a casualty is breathing, but unconscious.

An unconscious breathing casualty with suspected spinal injury should be left in the position found unless the airway is compromised. The airway can be maintained by turning the casualty with a modified recovery position technique – see Section 17.

Kneel beside the casualty, remove any spectacles or wristwatch and check their pockets.

Place the arm nearest to you at right angles to their body with the arm bent in the position it falls. Do not attempt to force the arm into an unnatural position.

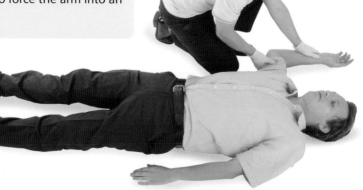

Bring the arm furthest away from you across the chest and hold the back of the hand against the nearest cheek.

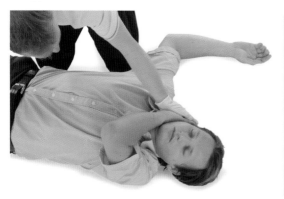

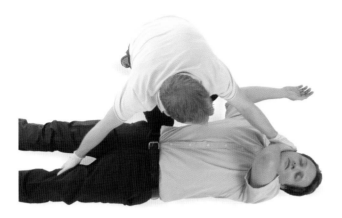

With your other hand, grasp the far leg just above the knee and pull it up but keep the foot on the ground.

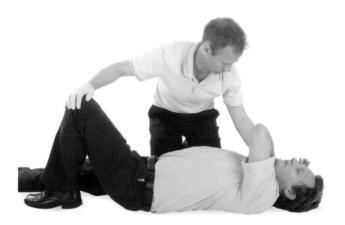

Keep their hand pressed against the cheek and pull on the leg to roll the casualty towards you and onto their side.

Roll gently, supporting the head constantly.

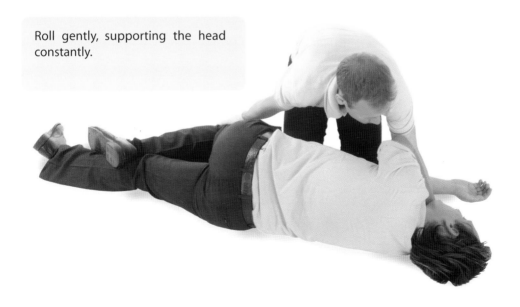

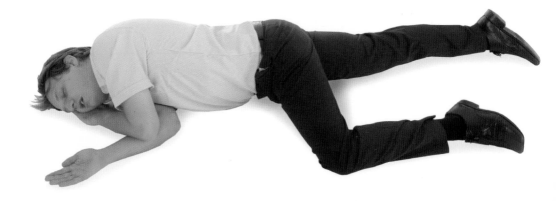

Adjust the upper leg so that both the hip and knee are bent at right angles. Tilt the head back to make sure the airway remains open. Adjust the hand under the cheek if necessary to keep the head tilted.

Recheck the airway.

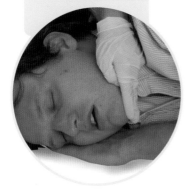

Recheck the airway and breathing and call 999/112 for an ambulance if you have not already sent someone to make the call. Casualties should be placed injured-side down if possible. Heavily pregnant casualties should be placed on their left-hand side if injuries allow. This alleviates pressure on the deep veins returning blood from the womb. If the casualty is already lying on their front or side you can manoeuvre them into a recovery position without having to turn them. Keep the casualty warm and monitor them constantly. The casualty should not be left in the same position for more than 30 minutes. If injuries allow, turn them onto their other side.

Casualty in recovery position.

BREATHING & CIRCULATION

The air that we breathe and take for granted is made up of numerous gases, in particular:

○ Nitrogen 79%
○ Oxygen 20.4%
○ Carbon Dioxide and others 0.6%

Oxygen is essential to maintain and support life. Without it our vital organs can only survive for a few minutes.

THE BREATHING PROCESS

We are able to breathe in when our diaphragm contracts and flattens. At the same time the ribs are elevated. As negative pressure is produced in the chest cavity there is increased pressure in the abdomen. Air is drawn into the lungs to equalize the pressure. This takes place when the levels of carbon dioxide in the blood rise to stimulate the respiratory centre of the brain into sending messages to the muscles of the diaphragm and chest. We exhale when the diaphragm relaxes and the chest wall and lung tissue return to their original size.

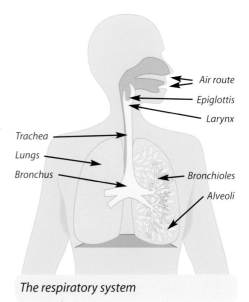

The respiratory system

Air can only enter the lungs via the airways. This is composed of the nasal passage and mouth. From here, air travels into the trachea (windpipe). The windpipe begins at the lower end of the larynx (voice box) and ends by dividing into the left and right bronchi. The bronchi are the branches of the trachea that carry air to the smaller elements of the lungs known as the bronchioles and alveoli.

There are more than 200 million alveoli in the lungs that have tiny blood capillaries in their membrane. When air enters the lungs, it comes into contact with these capillaries and filters through to create an exchange of oxygen into the blood stream and at the same time returning carbon dioxide into the alveoli to be exhaled.

These capillaries allow the oxygenated blood to pass into the pulmonary vein where it is transported to the heart. De-oxygenated blood containing carbon dioxide is carried back to the lungs from the heart via the pulmonary artery.

During the process of respiration we use approximately 4% of the oxygen we breathe in. On expiration we breathe out carbon dioxide and approximately 16% oxygen.

The average breathing rate in an adult is approximately 10 - 16 breaths per minute.

THE PRINCIPLES OF RESUSCITATION

The term resuscitation, expired air ventilations (EAV) or rescue breathing can best be described as the restoration of life to someone who is unconscious and not breathing normally.

This is done by artificially moving air in and out of the lungs to provide a casualty with the necessary oxygen to maintain life.

The recognised methods for this action are either by mouth to mouth or mouth to nose. The method used will depend on which is most suitable in order to inflate the lungs. For example, if a casualty has suffered severe facial injuries or you have to resuscitate in water it may be necessary to inflate via the mouth to nose method.

During the resuscitation of a casualty it is essential to maintain:
○ The movement of air in and out of the lungs
○ The pumping of oxygenated blood to the vital parts of the body

If the heart has stopped beating, rescue breathing will not be sufficient. Rescue breathing combined with chest compressions will be required. This is known as Cardiopulmonary Resuscitation or CPR.

In cases where a person has had surgery for cancer of the larynx (voice box), sections of the airway may have been removed and they will breathe through a hole in the throat. This is often referred to as a stoma. Breathing takes place via the stoma instead of the mouth or nose.

During your checks for normal breathing you may hear air escaping from the neck area indicating that the casualty has a stoma fitted.

When resuscitating casualties with a stoma, you should open the airway as normal but close the mouth and nose and breathe directly into the stoma.

For the procedure that should be adopted when giving rescue breaths to a casualty with suspected spinal injuries see Section 17.

THE BASIC LIFE SUPPORT ACTION PLAN

To continue from the primary assessment where the aim was to establish if the casualty was responsive and breathing normally, we will now look at the action plan for Basic Life Support.

THE CASUALTY IS CONSCIOUS AND BREATHING NORMALLY
If the casualty is responsive but has suffered severe injuries, leave them in the position found and treat accordingly. Otherwise, establish the possible cause of the collapse, treat any injuries and obtain medical assistance if necessary.

THE CASUALTY IS UNCONSCIOUS AND BREATHING NORMALLY
If the casualty is breathing, check for any injuries and treat accordingly. Place your casualty in the recovery position. Obtain medical assistance. Monitor breathing and keep your casualty warm.

THE CASUALTY IS UNCONSCIOUS AND NOT BREATHING NORMALLY

Immediately send someone to call 999/112 for an ambulance.

Studies over recent years have shown that calling for the Emergency Services as soon as you determine the casualty is not breathing normally increases their chance of survival. If no help is available you should leave the casualty to call for an ambulance yourself. Upon returning to the casualty, recheck for safety, and start compressions immediately – 30 initially.

THE CASUALTY IS NOT BREATHING NORMALLY DUE TO INJURY OR DROWNING

In this case, breathing will have ceased because of breathing difficulties rather than a medical condition. If you are on your own you should call for an ambulance immediately. Upon returning to the casualty, re-check for safety, and start CPR
i.e. 30:2. (Compressions : Breaths).

LIFEGUARDS

If your casualty has drowned and you are a qualified lifeguard you must perform CPR for 1 minute before calling the emergency services i.e. 5 initial breaths, 30 chest compressions, 2 breaths, 30 chest compressions, 2 breaths.

If you are not a lifeguard, then the standard Basic Life Support protocols must be applied, i.e. if your casualty is not breathing, you must call for the emergency services immediately. Or send your bystander if you have one. Upon your return you must start CPR - 30 compressions to 2 breaths and continue until medical assistance arrives and tells you to stop, you become exhausted, or the casualty starts breathing.

BASIC LIFE SUPPORT

Carry out the procedures for your primary assessment. If the casualty is not already on their back turn them over, open their airway and check for normal breathing for up to 10 seconds. If your casualty is not breathing normally call 999/112 then start CPR immeadiately.

CARDIOPULMONARY RESUSCITATION (CPR)

Chest compressions are performed with the casualty lying on their back on a firm surface.

By depressing the chest, oxygenated blood is forced out of the heart and around the body.

○ Kneel by the side of the casualty
○ Place the heel of one hand in the centre of the casualty's chest

Place your other hand on top of the first hand with the fingers interlocked. Straighten your arms and bring your shoulders over the centre of the casualty's chest.

Interlock the fingers.

Use the heel and palm of your hands to compress the chest. Keep your fingers clear of pressing down over the ribcage. Do not apply any pressure over the upper abdomen or bottom end of the breastbone.

Compress the chest 30 times at a depth of 4-5 cm and at a rate of 100 compressions per minute. After each compression release all the pressure from the chest without losing contact between your hands and the sternum (breastbone). Compressions and release should take equal amounts of time.

A good chest compression should be to a depth of 4 to 5 centimetres.

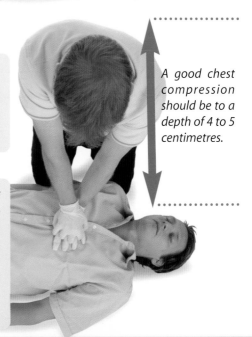

Immediately follow the 30 compressions with 2 rescue breaths. Continue this action until the emergency services take over. Another trained person can take over if you become too exhausted to continue.

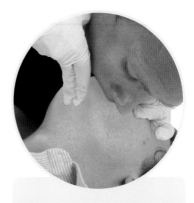

The action of CPR is unlikely to restart the heart for the vast majority of your casualties. However, it is essential to ensure that oxygenated blood is pumped to the vital organs in order to offer your casualty some form of life support.

Therefore, it is important to continue with your Basic Life Support procedures, i.e. 30 chest compressions to 2 breaths.

Remember to give 2 effective rescue breaths.

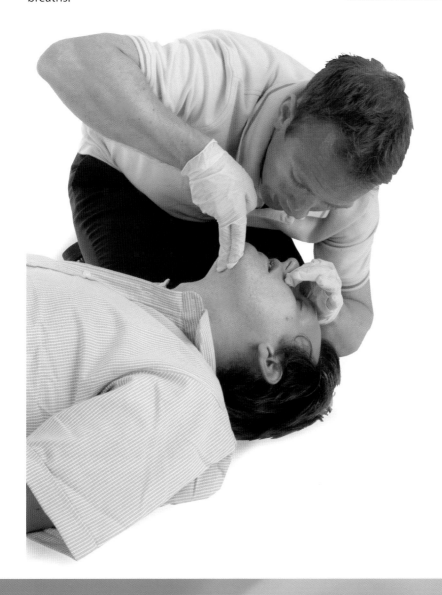

FIRST AID at work

THE CHAIN OF SURVIVAL

To prevent Cardiac Arrest	To buy time	To restart the heart	To restore quality of life

EARLY RECOGNITION & CALL FOR HELP

Dial 999/112 when the casualty is not breathing

EARLY CPR

Start CPR to buy time until medical help arrives

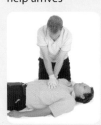

EARLY DEFIBRILLATION

Defibrillators give an electric shock to reorganize the rhythm of the heart

Photo courtesy of ZOLL Medical U.K.Ltd

POST RESUSCITATION CARE

Care provided by the paramedics and the hospital

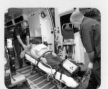

Photo courtesy of ZOLL Medical U.K.Ltd

GIVE 2 EFFECTIVE RESCUE BREATHS

- After 30 compressions open the airway again using head tilt and chin lift.
- Pinch the soft part of the casualty's nose closed, using your index finger and thumb of your hand on his forehead.
- Allow the casualty's mouth to open, but maintain chin lift.
- Take a normal breath and place your lips around the casualty's mouth, making sure that you have a good seal.
- Blow steadily into the casualty's mouth whilst watching for the chest to rise; take about one second to make sure the casualty's chest rises as in normal breathing; this is an effective rescue breath.
- Maintaining head tilt and chin lift, take your mouth away from the casualty and watch for the chest to fall as air passes out.
- Take another normal breath and blow into the casualty's mouth once more to give a total of two effective rescue breaths. Then return your hands without delay to the correct position on the sternum and give a further 30 chest compressions.
- Continue with chest compressions and rescue breaths in a ratio of 30:2.
- Stop to recheck the casualty only if they start breathing normally; otherwise **do not interrupt resuscitation.**

If your rescue breaths do not make the chest rise as in normal breathing, then before your next attempt:
- Check the casualty's mouth and remove any obstruction.
- Recheck there is adequate head tilt and chin lift.
- Do not attempt more than two breaths each time before returning to chest compressions.

If there is more than one rescuer present, another should take over CPR every 1-2 min to prevent fatigue. Ensure the minimum of delay during the changeover of rescuers.

Chest-compression-only CPR:
- If you are not able or are unwilling to give rescue breaths, give chest compression only.
- If chest compressions only are given, these should be continuous at a rate of 100 per minute.
- Stop to recheck the casualty only if he starts breathing normally; otherwise **do not interrupt resuscitation.**

RESUSCITATION AND CROSS INFECTION

The Resuscitation Council UK state that rescue breathing by means of mouth to mouth, or nose methods carries little or no risk of infection from AIDS. For hygiene purposes you may wish to use a resuscitation face shield or pocket mask if you have been trained in how to use them correctly.

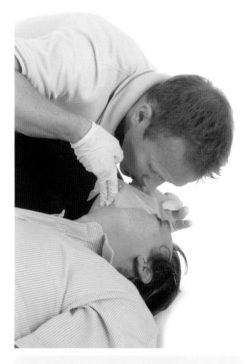

Resuscitation using a face shield.

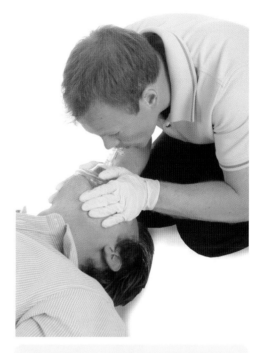

Resuscitation using a pocket mask.

RESUSCITATION DURING PREGNANCY

During the final weeks of pregnancy, or if the woman is pregnant with more than one baby there is increased pressure on the stomach, diaphragm and lungs. A modified approach to resuscitation is required at this time.

If the pregnant woman is unconscious and breathing she should be turned onto her left-hand side to clear and open her airway.

For resuscitation, padding is needed under her right buttock to tilt her slightly to the left. This is known as the Left Lateral Tilt technique as it effectively moves the weight of the baby off the mother's deep veins allowing effective movement of blood back to the heart.

Chest compressions should be carried out as normal but the First Aider should adjust their own position to ensure they are correctly aligned on the breastbone.

ADULT BASIC LIFE SUPPORT

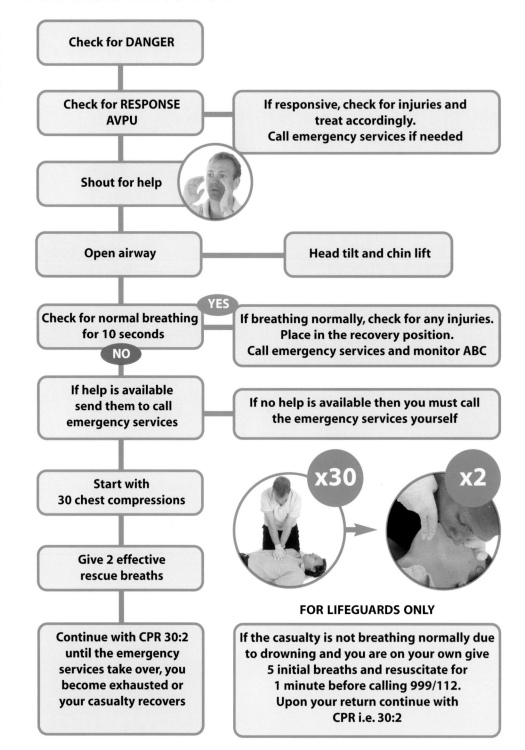

Check for DANGER

Check for RESPONSE AVPU

If responsive, check for injuries and treat accordingly.
Call emergency services if needed

Shout for help

Open airway

Head tilt and chin lift

Check for normal breathing for 10 seconds

YES — If breathing normally, check for any injuries. Place in the recovery position. Call emergency services and monitor ABC

NO

If help is available send them to call emergency services

If no help is available then you must call the emergency services yourself

Start with 30 chest compressions

Give 2 effective rescue breaths

x30   x2

FOR LIFEGUARDS ONLY

Continue with CPR 30:2 until the emergency services take over, you become exhausted or your casualty recovers

If the casualty is not breathing normally due to drowning and you are on your own give 5 initial breaths and resuscitate for 1 minute before calling 999/112. Upon your return continue with CPR i.e. 30:2

SECTION SUMMARY

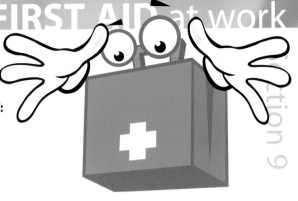

ACTIONS THAT SHOULD BE TAKEN WHEN CARRYING OUT A PRIMARY ASSESSMENT:
- Check for danger
- Check for a response
- Shout for help
- Open the airway
- Check for normal breathing

IF A CASUALTY IS CONSCIOUS AND BREATHING NORMALLY YOU SHOULD:
- Carry out a secondary assessment to check for any injuries or medical conditions and treat accordingly. If necessary call for an ambulance.

IF A CASUALTY IS UNCONSCIOUS BUT BREATHING NORMALLY YOU SHOULD:
- Carry out a secondary assessment to check for any injuries or medical conditions and treat accordingly. Place the casualty in the recovery position and call for an ambulance.

AN UNCONSCIOUS NORMAL BREATHING CASUALTY IS PUT INTO THE RECOVERY POSITION TO:
- Maintain an open and clear airway
- Allow fluids to drain from the mouth
- Keep the casualty comfortable
- Aid normal breathing.

IF A CASUALTY IS UNCONSCIOUS AND NOT BREATHING NORMALLY YOU SHOULD:
- Immediately call for an ambulance if you are on your own or send a bystander to call for an ambulance immediately.
- Return to the casualty
- Start CPR 30 chest compressions followed by 2 breaths and continue until medical help tells you to stop, you become exhausted or your casualty recovers.

THE SPEED AND DEPTH OF CHEST COMPRESSIONS IS:
- 100 beats per minute at a depth of 4 to 5 cm.

LIFEGUARDS:
IF YOU ARE ON YOUR OWN AND DEALING WITH A CASUALTY WHO IS NOT BREATHING DUE TO DROWNING, YOU SHOULD:
- Give 5 initial rescue breaths
- Resuscitate or give CPR for 1 minute before calling for an ambulance.

DISORDERS OF RESPIRATION

When oxygen cannot reach the tissues of the body due to an obstruction or damage to the respiratory system, the term asphyxia is generally used to describe this action. The vital organs of the body can only survive for a few minutes without oxygen so the need to remove any obstruction or provide rescue breaths to a casualty is vital.

MAIN CAUSES OF ASPHYXIA

Paralysis of the respiratory nervous system	Electrocution, poisoning, drug abuse, head injury, spinal cord damage in the neck
Compression to the chest	Sand or earth, damage to the chest wall caused by car steering wheel impact
Lack of oxygen in the air	Motor exhaust fumes, carbon monoxide, smoke filled rooms, change in atmospheric pressure from high altitude or deep sea diving
Compression of the neck	Hanging or strangulation, damage caused by an injury to the face and neck restricting airflow
Suffocation and obstructed airway	Drowning, a pillow or plastic bag over the face, vomit or bodily fluids, choking, asthma, severe allergic reaction
Medical conditions	Damage to the lungs from an injury, lung infection and disorders, unconsciousness

Without the vital supply of oxygen, blood will return from the lungs to the heart with very little or a complete depletion of oxygen.

This low level of oxygen in the blood and tissues is known as hypoxia.

With certain medical conditions such as asthma and other respiratory disorders that may cause a partial obstruction of the airway, the signs and symptoms of hypoxia may be mild at first with rapid progression as the condition deteriorates.

RECOGNITION OF HYPOXIA

- ○ Distressed rapid breathing becoming noisy
- ○ Pale, grey/blue skin affecting the nails, lips, eyelids and ears at first, with the whole body being affected as the condition worsens. This is known as cyanosis
- ○ Distress and anxiety
- ○ Confusion
- ○ Nausea
- ○ Aggression
- ○ Weakness

TREATMENT FOR HYPOXIA

- ○ Ensure that the area is safe for you to approach
- ○ Treat the cause
- ○ Maintain the airway and breathing
- ○ Dial 999/112 for an ambulance

If the condition is not reversed, hypoxia will lead to unconsciousness and a cessation of breathing.

You will also see the signs and symptoms of hypoxia in conditions that reduce the amount of oxygenated blood carried around the body. These will be covered in more detail in Section 11.

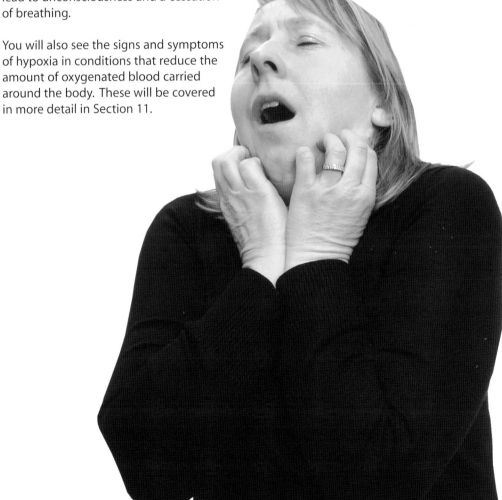

Section 10

AIRWAY OBSTRUCTION AND BREATHING DISORDERS

The respiratory system comprising of the nose, mouth, trachea (windpipe), bronchus, bronchioles and alveoli are all in complete communication with each other as long as there are no obstructions.

Severe breathing difficulties can take place when the process of normal breathing is affected. This can be caused by a medical condition or illness, emotional and physical shock, anxiety or when the airway becomes partially or fully obstructed.

CAUSES
- Foreign objects
- Blood, vomit or water
- Smoke inhalation
- Burns to the face and neck
- Severe allergic reactions
- Injuries to the face and neck
- Asthma
- Hyperventilation
- Emotional or physical shock
- Chest and abdominal injury

RECOGNITION
- The signs and symptoms of hypoxia
- Difficulty in speaking
- Distressed, noisy breathing
- Flaring of the nostrils
- Sucking in of the chest wall and ribs
- Coughing
- Coughed-up blood
- Difficulty in breathing out

Whatever the cause, a casualty will need to be treated immediately
- If possible, remove any obstruction
- Restore and maintain normal breathing
- Calm, reassure and monitor
- Seek medical attention even if they recover
- If unconscious and breathing place them in the recovery position and call 999/112

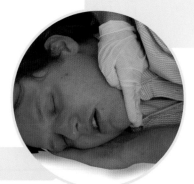

Recheck the airway.

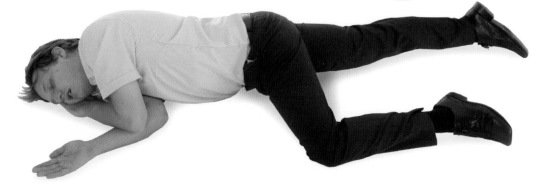

Casualty in recovery position.

CHOKING

A foreign object that becomes stuck in the throat or windpipe may cause a partial or full blockage. This could also lead to spasms of the muscles in the upper airway.

The casualty can often clear a partial obstruction if you encourage them to cough and remain calm.

A full obstruction will need urgent attention with rescue breaths and chest compressions if the casualty becomes unconscious and stops breathing.

RECOGNITION
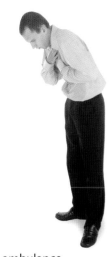
- Evidence of what may have caused the obstruction
- Casualty grasping at their throat
- Difficulty in speaking and breathing
- Congestion of the face and neck at first
- Pale grey/blue skin developing
- Anxiety and distress
- Weakness
- Becoming unconscious

TREATMENT OF A PARTIAL OBSTRUCTION FOR ADULTS
The casualty will be able to breathe and speak.
- Encourage the casualty to cough
- Calm and reassure
- Have them adopt a comfortable position
- If there is no improvement within 5 minutes call 999/112 for an ambulance
- Continually encourage the casualty to cough, and monitor their condition

TREATMENT OF A FULL OBSTRUCTION FOR ADULTS
The casualty will be unable to breathe or speak.
They will become weak and lose consciousness within minutes.

**ENCOURAGE THE CASUALTY TO COUGH
CHECK THE MOUTH AND REMOVE
ANY OBSTRUCTIONS**

Lean the casualty forward and support the upper chest with one hand. Stand behind the casualty and give sharp slaps between the shoulder blades.
DO THIS UP TO 5 TIMES.
Check the mouth and remove any obstructions.

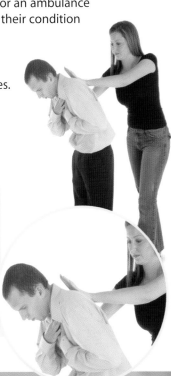

Give up to 5 back slaps.

If the back slaps are unsuccessful, stand behind the casualty and place both arms around them, lean the casualty forwards. Place one fist just below the breastbone on the upper abdomen and grasp the fist fully with your other hand. Pull sharply inwards and upwards to force the obstruction out.

DO THIS UP TO 5 TIMES.

Check the mouth and remove any obstructions.

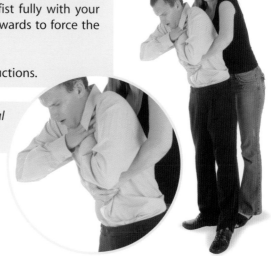

Give up to 5 abdominal thrusts.

Repeat the cycle of backslaps and abdominal thrusts 3 times. If the obstruction has not cleared call 999/112 for an ambulance and continue the procedure.

If at any time the casualty becomes unconscious, support the casualty to the ground and call for an ambulance immediately. Commence C.P.R. immediately (Section 9) i.e. 30 Chest compressions to 2 rescue breaths continuously.

SMOKE AND FUME INHALATION

The inhalation of smoke or toxic fumes from fires, solvent abuse or defective heating systems will lead to a lack of oxygen circulating around the body (hypoxia), burns to the airway and damage to the heart, lung tissue and blood.

Fires will burn up the available supply of oxygen in an enclosed space very quickly. A fire has many products of combustion some of which chemically displace oxygen from our blood. Carbon monoxide is a major product of combustion in many fires whilst domestic fires can produce hydrogen cyanide. Toxic fumes can do an enormous amount of damage to the lungs and blood and reduce the blood's ability to carry oxygen.

RECOGNITION
SMOKE
Low oxygen content, containing toxic fumes causing:
- Irritation and burning of the airway
- Sooty deposits around the mouth and nose
- Hypoxia
- Coughing
- Unconsciousness

CARBON DIOXIDE
An odourless, colourless gas that accumulates in enclosed spaces and displaces oxygen causing:
- Breathlessness
- Headache
- Weakness
- Unconsciousness

CARBON MONOXIDE
A colourless gas produced in natural gas, coal and exhaust fumes causing:
- Headache
- Nausea
- Confusion
- Difficulty in breathing
- Skin to become cherry red in colour

SOLVENTS
Lighter fuels, glues, paint strippers, camping gas, cleaning fluids causing:
- Headache
- Vomiting
- Irritation of the airway and lungs
- Sudden cardiac arrest in some instances

TREATMENT
- If possible remove casualties into the fresh air
- Check airway and breathing
- Treat any burns and monitor the casualty's condition
- Treat unconscious casualties as normal and be prepared to resuscitate

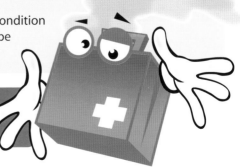

DO NOT ATTEMPT TO ENTER A BURNING OR SMOKE-FILLED AREA AS IT WILL PUT YOUR LIFE IN DANGER

DROWNING

Drowning is asphyxia caused by immersion in water but contrary to popular belief only a small amount of water enters the lungs. In the initial stages of drowning there will be a reflex spasm of the larynx. This will close the airway not allowing any water to enter the lungs. Eventually this reflex action relaxes and water enters the lungs thus resulting in WET DROWNING. In some cases the larynx remains closed, blocking the airway. This happens when extreme fear or panic takes over after someone finds themselves out of their depth or having fallen into deep water. This is known as DRY DROWNING.

In nearly all cases of drowning, a small amount of water will enter the lungs causing an irritation and a build-up of fluid in the lungs. This will interfere with the transfer of oxygen into the blood stream. This process can take up to 72 hours to develop and is known as SECONDARY DROWNING.

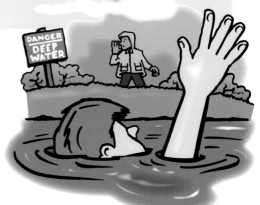

RECOGNITION
- The casualty may be face down in the water or completely submerged
- Water flowing from the casualty's mouth when recovering
- Vomiting
- Signs and symptoms of hypoxia
- Coughing
- Unconscious with no breathing

TREATMENT
- Only enter the water if you are capable and trained to perform water rescues. Try reaching the casualty with a pole or rope
- Get the casualty's head above the water and keep them horizontal
- Recover to land and clear the airway
- Open the airway and check for breathing
- If unconscious but breathing, place them in the recovery position with the body raised slightly higher than the head. This will allow water to drain from the stomach naturally
- Do not force the water out as this will induce vomiting
- If your casualty stops breathing you must call 999/112 immediately even if you are on your own. Return to your casualty and start C.P.R. i.e. 30 chest compressions to 2 breaths continuously
- Continue with this procedure until the casualty recovers or the paramedics take over or you become exhausted
- Treat all drowning victims for hypothermia if necessary
- Resuscitation of drowning victims can be difficult at first due to water in the lungs and the effects of cold. There will be increased resistance when giving rescue breaths and chest compressions
- All victims of drowning should be sent to hospital even if they appear to make a full recovery
- If the casualty has an epileptic seizure in water, treat as for drowning and send them to hospital as water may have entered the lungs during the seizure

HYPERVENTILATION

Hyperventilation is when the breathing rate is greatly increased leading to an imbalance of oxygen and carbon dioxide in the blood. This is often caused by severe stress, anxiety, fear and panic. There may also be an underlying medical condition causing the problem. In some cases with both children and adults, hyperventilation can be used as an attention seeking ploy.

RECOGNITION
- Rapid and shallow breathing
- Feeling of being light-headed or dizzy
- Tingling in the fingers and toes
- Muscle cramps in the hands and feet
- Anxiety and the feeling of being unable to breathe

TREATMENT
- If the cause is due to a panic attack or anxiety, remove the casualty to a quiet place. Advise them to breathe at a slower rate and do this by counting the rate and reducing it
- If this has no effect, encourage them to breathe into their cupped hands or a paper bag. The casualty will re-breathe their expired air which will help to increase the low levels of carbon dioxide.

The use of re-breathing into a paper bag should be used as a last resort. Monitor the casualty very closely as this can cause an adverse reaction with some casualties.

- If hyperventilation has been brought on by an injury, poisoning or a medical condition, seek urgent medical advice

If there is no improvement in the condition call 999/112 for an ambulance

ASTHMA

Asthma is a very serious medical condition affecting the smaller air passages of the respiratory system. Muscle spasms and an increased production of mucus cause the airways to become narrowed and inflamed. Many people die as a result of asthma attacks each year. There are numerous factors or triggers that bring on an asthma attack. Colds, infections, allergic reactions, changes in temperature, exercise and stress are the most common. Asthma sufferers are usually prescribed medications that help to prevent attacks. These are commonly colour coded in shades of red, brown and gold. Medications for the relief of asthma during an attack are commonly coded in shades of blue or grey.

RECOGNITION
○ Breathlessness and difficulty in speaking
○ Difficulty in breathing out, sometimes wheezing
○ Coughing
○ Breathing out may be slow and prolonged
○ Increased breathing effort
○ Signs and symptoms of hypoxia with blueness at the lips and extremities. The casualty will become weaker as the attack becomes acute.

TREATMENT
○ Help the casualty to a comfortable sitting position
○ Calm and reassure them
○ Encourage them to use their own prescribed medication
○ If their reliever medication has no effect, if the attack lasts for more than 5 minutes or if this is the first attack, call 999/112 for an ambulance
○ If the casualty becomes unconscious, carry out your Basic Life Support procedures

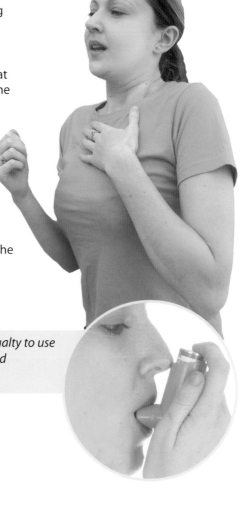

Encourage the casualty to use their own prescribed medication.

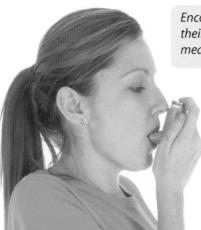

SECTION SUMMARY

WHAT IS ASPHYXIA?
○ When oxygen is prevented from entering the body

WHAT IS HYPOXIA?
○ Low level of oxygen in the blood

WHAT CAN CAUSE ASPHYXIA?
○ Choking
○ Suffocation
○ Crushed chest
○ Strangulation
○ Drowning
○ Anaphylactic shock
○ Convulsions
○ High altitude

HOW SHOULD YOU TREAT SOMEBODY WHO IS CHOKING?
○ Encourage to cough. Give up to 5 backslaps, followed by up to 5 abdominal thrusts. Repeat 3 times and call Emergency Services if the obstruction is still there. Be prepared to resuscitate. (See next section for more detail)

HOW SHOULD YOU TREAT AN ASTHMA ATTACK?
○ Sit the casualty down and encourage them to use their reliever inhaler. If this does not work or they do not have an inhaler call for an ambulance.
(See next section for more detail)

WHAT EFFECT WILL SMOKE OR TOXIC FUME INHALATION HAVE ON THE AIRWAY?
○ Causes burning and swelling of the airway

HOW SHOULD YOU TREAT HYPERVENTILATION?
○ Calm the casualty. Sit them down and encourage to breathe slowly. Get them to breathe into their cupped hands

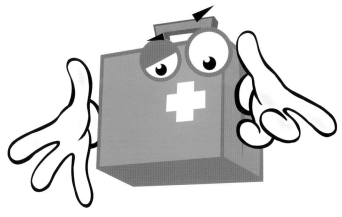

THE CIRCULATORY SYSTEM

The heart is a muscular pump a little larger than a clenched fist. Its primary purpose is to pump 24 hours a day, 60 to 80 times a minute in the case of an adult. With each beat the heart pumps blood that delivers life-sustaining oxygen and nutrients to 300 trillion cells. Each day the average heart 'beats' 100,000 times and pumps about 2,000 gallons of blood. In a 70-year lifetime an average human heart beats more than 2.5 billion times. The circulatory system is a network of flexible tubes through which blood flows as it carries oxygen and nutrients to all parts of the body. This includes the heart, lungs, arteries, arterioles (small arteries), capillaries (minute blood vessels), veins and venules (small veins). Oxygenated blood is pumped from the left side of the heart to the body via the arteries. De-oxygenated blood is transported back to the heart via the veins, which is then pumped from the right side of the heart to the lungs to collect more oxygen. The average adult has approximately 6 litres of blood which is composed of 55% plasma (of which 90% is water), red cells, white cells and platelets.

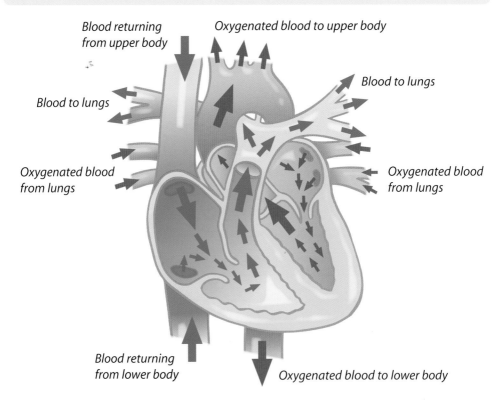

Blood returning from upper body

Oxygenated blood to upper body

Blood to lungs

Blood to lungs

Oxygenated blood from lungs

Oxygenated blood from lungs

Blood returning from lower body

Oxygenated blood to lower body

The blood vessels within this system are the:

ARTERIES Deliver oxygenated blood from the heart to the body. They have strong flexible walls

VEINS Allow the blood to flow back to the heart by the action of muscles upon the thin walls. One-way valves keep the flow directed towards the heart

CAPILLARIES These small, sometimes microscopic vessels form a link between the arteries, veins and body tissue. This allows the transfer of oxygen, and nutrients to the body, and the waste products to be removed

THE COMPOSITION OF BLOOD
- **Red cells**   Carry haemoglobin that binds with oxygen
- **White cells**   Help fight infection
- **Plasma**   The fluid component of the blood
- **Platelets**   Aid the blood to clot

The pulse is a pressure wave that is felt as the heart contracts and pumps blood through the arteries. It is felt where an artery passes close to the surface of the body.

THE PULSE
- **Carotid**   In the neck
- **Radial**   In the wrist
- **Brachial**   In the inside of the upper arm

Although the pulse is no longer checked when looking for signs of circulation for a non-breathing casualty, it is beneficial to be able to recognise a pulse for a breathing casualty with various medical conditions or injuries. This can act as an indicator of improvement or deterioration.

To check for a pulse use your fingertips not your thumb as it has its own pulse. Feel for the rate per minute, the strength and the rhythm. The average adult pulse rate is between 60 and 80 beats per minute.

What can go wrong with the circulatory system?
- Blood loss – obviously the more blood we lose the less there is available to sustain the vital organs. Any loss greater than 0.5 litres will have an effect upon the body
- Loss of body fluids – severe diarrhoea and vomiting, burns and dehydration
- Heart disorders – heart attack or angina
- Fainting
- Anaphylactic shock
- Poisoning or substance abuse

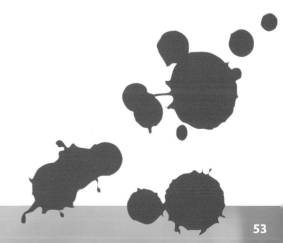

SHOCK

Shock is best described as circulatory failure or collapse when the arterial blood pressure is too low to provide an adequate supply of blood to the tissues. As a result of this, the vital organs such as the heart and brain are deprived of oxygen.

Shock can be brought on by:
○ A severe loss of blood from internal and external bleeding
○ Loss of bodily fluid due to burns
○ Excessive vomiting and diarrhoea
○ A reduced blood supply or activity of the heart as with a heart attack or coronary thrombosis
○ Widespread dilation of the veins with insufficient blood to fill them. This can be caused by bacteria or chemical toxins
○ Injury to the spinal cord
○ Severe head trauma that damages the nerves controlling circulation
○ Changes in blood pressure

Emotional shock is an over stimulation of the vagus nerve. Pain, fright and emotional distress can cause this. With this type of shock the blood pressure is lowered.

RECOGNITION
○ Pale, blue/grey, cold and clammy skin
○ Rapid but weak pulse
○ Weak and confused
○ Nausea and thirst
○ Rapid shallow breathing as the condition deteriorates
○ Unconsciousness

TREATMENT
○ Treat the cause (bleeding, burns or injuries)
○ If injuries allow, lay the casualty down
○ Raise and support the legs but be aware of injuries to the spine and legs
○ Loosen tight clothing
○ Keep the casualty warm with blankets or coats
○ Insulate from the ground
○ Call 999/112 for an ambulance. Calm and reassure
○ Monitor the casualty's airway and breathing
○ Do not let them have anything to eat, drink or smoke
○ If they become unconscious follow your Basic Life Support procedures.

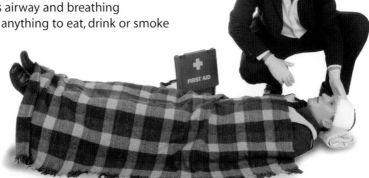

OTHER METHODS OF TREATING SHOCK

If the casualty is in shock but suffering from a breathing problem or a heart disorder:
- Lay the casualty down
- Raise the head and shoulders
- Bend the knees
- Place support under the knees and behind the back

If the casualty is in shock but suffering with injuries that do not allow you to raise the legs:
- Lay the casualty down
- Slightly bend and support the knees to aid circulation procedures

FAINTING

Fainting is a brief loss of consciousness caused by a sudden lack of oxygenated blood reaching the brain. This is often caused by an emotional reaction, lack of food or drink, exhaustion, pain or fear. Another cause is prolonged periods of having to stand without any movement causing the blood to pool in the legs. This causes a reduction in the amount of oxygenated blood circulating normally to the brain.

RECOGNITION
- Pale, cold and clammy skin
- Sudden but normally brief unconsciousness
- Slow pulse
- Nausea and sometimes vomiting

TREATMENT
- If a casualty feels faint advise them to lie down
- Raise their legs about the height of the chest in order to circulate blood towards the heart and brain
- If the casualty has fainted and fallen, check for any injuries and treat accordingly
- Do not let bystanders crowd the casualty and ensure that they have plenty of fresh air
- If the casualty has a heart condition, a head injury or suffered a stroke do not raise the legs because the increased blood flow will cause complications
- Fainting is normally brief. If the casualty faints repreatedly or they do not regain consciousness there may be an underlying cause, so call 999/112 for an ambulance
- Monitor the casualty's airway and breathing and be prepared to carry out the procedures for Basic Life Support

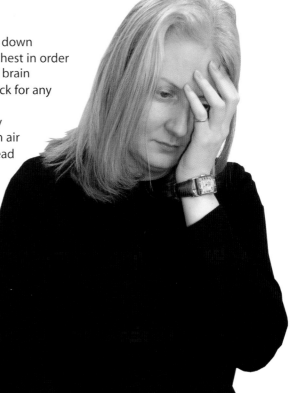

HEART ATTACK

A heart attack is one of the most common of numerous heart conditions that will require life saving First Aid. A heart attack, which is known as a myocardial infarction occurs when there is a blockage in one of the coronary arteries that supply the heart muscle with oxygenated blood. If part of the heart does not receive oxygenated blood, the heart muscle will die or not function correctly, reducing the amount of blood pumped around the body. The severity of the attack depends on the location of the blockage. If the blockage is in one of the smaller blood vessels it will cause the casualty to have chest pain and other signs and symptoms. This is treatable and a recovery is made after medical treatment. The blockage of a major blood vessel may lead to sudden collapse and cardiac arrest.

RECOGNITION
○ Central chest pain radiating between the abdomen and the jaw
  and possibly down one arm
○ A crushing, restricting feeling on and around the chest
○ Rapid breathing and a shortness of breath
○ Rapid or irregular pulse
○ Pale, cold and clammy skin with a blue/grey appearance
○ Nausea and vomiting and a feeling of severe indigestion

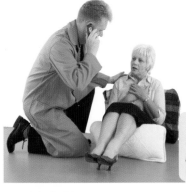

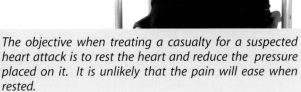

The objective when treating a casualty for a suspected heart attack is to rest the heart and reduce the pressure placed on it. It is unlikely that the pain will ease when rested.

TREATMENT
○ Assist the casualty to rest. This should be in a comfortable position, generally a half-sitting position with support for head, back and under the knees
○ Call 999/112 for an ambulance
○ Monitor the casualty's airway and breathing
○ Loosen any tight restricting clothing
○ Calm and reassure
○ Keep them warm but do not overheat
○ If the casualty becomes unconscious carry out your procedure for Basic Life Support

ADMINISTERING ASPRIN TO A CASUALTY

The administration of an Asprin to a casualty suffering a heart attack has proved to be a benefit, as it slows down the clotting process. However, some people are allergic to Asprin. Only adminster Asprin if you know for sure that your casualty is not allergic to it.

If in doubt DO NOT ADMINISTER.

DO NOT KEEP ASPRIN IN YOUR FIRST AID KIT.

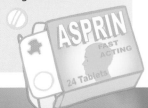

ANGINA PECTORIS

An angina attack occurs when there is a narrowing of the coronary artery. This can be either by a build-up of fatty deposits or a collapsed arterial wall making it difficult for blood to flow freely to the heart. An attack may occur during exertion or stress. Most angina sufferers are prescribed medication in the form of a spray or tablets. This helps to relax the walls of the blood vessels allowing blood to flow.

RECOGNITION
○ Initially the signs and symptoms will be the same as a heart attack
○ Sudden weakness, fear and anxiety
○ Evidence of exertion, exercise or stress
○ Signs and symptoms will ease with rest

TREATMENT
○ Rest the casualty as for a heart attack
○ Encourage them to use their medication
○ If the pain does not ease with rest, or if it is their first attack, treat as a heart attack and call 999/112 for an ambulance

WHAT IS THE MAIN DIFFERENCE BETWEEN A HEART ATTACK AND AN ANGINA ATTACK?
○ An angina attack will ease with rest
○ An angina sufferer may have medication for their condition

ANAPHYLACTIC SHOCK

Anaphylactic shock is a severe allergic reaction causing the body to produce large quantities of histamine. This can lead to swelling or constriction of the airways and widening of the blood vessels leading to circulatory collapse and heart failure. There are numerous triggers for this reaction including food (peanuts, dairy products, wheat), medicines (aspirin), chemicals and insect stings. Sufferers of severe allergic reactions are often prescribed medication to relieve the condition. Medication is usually an Epipen, containing adrenaline, for self-injection or it may be in tablet form.

RECOGNITION
○ Anxiety
○ Swelling of the face and neck
○ Swelling of the mouth and tongue
○ Red blotchy skin
○ Difficulty in breathing and wheezing
○ Rapid pulse
○ Signs and symptoms of shock

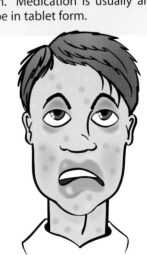

TREATMENT
○ Call 999/112 for an ambulance
○ Sit the casualty up if they are conscious
○ Encourage the casualty to use medication if available
○ Be prepared to open the airway and resuscitate
○ Monitor the casualty's airway and breathing
○ Even if the casualty appears to recover they must be sent to hospital

SECTION SUMMARY

WHAT IS THE PURPOSE OF THE RESPIRATORY SYSTEM?
○ To take oxygen from the air we breathe and pass it into the circulatory system

WHAT MAKES UP THE CIRCULATORY SYSTEM?
○ Heart
○ Arteries
○ Veins
○ Capillaries
○ Blood

WHAT DO ARTERIES CARRY AROUND THE BODY?
○ Oxygenated blood

WHAT IS MEDICAL SHOCK?
○ A failure of the circulatory system leading to a drop in arterial blood pressure

HOW WOULD YOU RECOGNISE SHOCK?
○ Pale, cold, clammy skin
○ Rapid weak pulse
○ Rapid shallow breathing
○ Hypoxia
○ Confusion
○ Dizziness
○ Thirst
○ Nausea

HOW SHOULD YOU TREAT SHOCK?
○ Treat the cause
○ Lay the casualty down and raise the legs if injuries allow
○ Keep the casualty warm
○ Calm and reassure
○ Call for an ambulance

WHAT IS A HEART ATTACK?
○ A blockage of one or more of the coronary arteries

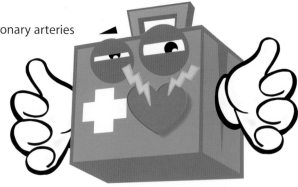

WOUNDS AND BLEEDING

A wound can be a break or opening in the surface of the skin which is often referred to as an open wound. When bleeding occurs internally it is known as a closed wound. Apart from the loss of blood which will lead to shock, there is the risk of infection. The infection could be caused by germs or cross-infection from the First Aider to the casualty and vice versa if hygiene precautions are not observed. Dealing with wounds can be unpleasant particularly with major bleeding but it must be remembered that unless treatment is carried out promptly and effectively the casualty's condition will deteriorate rapidly.

INCISED
A clean cut from a sharp edge that may be deep causing injury to underlying blood vessels or tissue, resulting in severe blood loss.

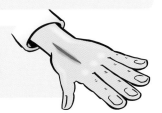

LACERATION
A rough tear or crush that is often harder to treat as the skin will be torn in more than one place. This wound carries a greater risk of infection.

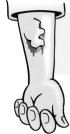

ABRASION
A graze or superficial wound from a rough surface with less bleeding but a high risk of infection.

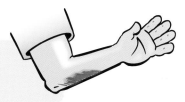

CONTUSION
A bruise or interal bleeding with damage to the capillaries under the skin. If the cause is severe there may be extensive internal bleeding.

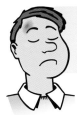

PUNCTURE
An object entering the body may cause   extensive damage to internal organs and infection will be carried inside the body.

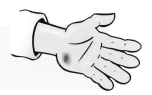

VELOCITY INJURY
A puncture wound at velocity will cause extensive damage to bones and internal organs leading to internal and external bleeding. There may be an exit wound which could be larger than the entry wound.

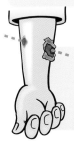

TYPES OF BLEEDING

BLEEDING FROM ARTERIES
This will pump from the wound in time with the heartbeat and is bright red in colour. Bleeding from a major artery will lead to shock, unconsciousness and death within minutes.

BLEEDING FROM VEINS
The blood will gush from the wound or pool at the site of the wound. This will depend on the size of the vein that has been damaged. The blood will be dark red in colour due to the oxygen being depleted.

BLEEDING FROM CAPILLARIES
Oozing at the site as with an abrasion or maybe internally from a contusion to muscle tissue and internal organs.

When a blood vessel is torn or severed, blood loss and shock cause the blood pressure to fall and the injured vessel to contract at the site of injury.

Platelets and proteins come into contact with the injured site and plug the wound. This process begins within ten minutes if the loss of blood is brought under control.

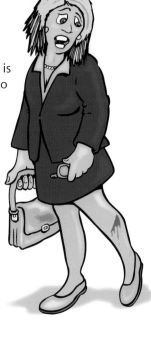

PREVENTING CROSS-INFECTION

Before treating a casualty for bleeding you should always think of safety and observe personal protection and hygiene control.
- ○ Wear disposable gloves
- ○ Where possible wash hands before dressing a wound
- ○ Cover cuts and grazes on your hands
- ○ Avoid touching the wound
- ○ Try not to talk, sneeze or cough over the wound
- ○ Place all soiled dressings and materials including gloves in a suitably marked (yellow) plastic bag
- ○ Put sharp items such as needles or syringes in containers for disposal

There is always the risk of cross-infection when dealing with bodily fluids. Blood borne viruses such as Hepatitis B and C and HIV can be contracted when the blood of an infected person comes into contact with an open sore, graze or wound of the First Aider.

CLINICAL WASTE

A safe approach and assessment must always take priority. The wearing of disposable gloves and the use of a resuscitation face shield or mask will help to eliminate the threat. There have been no reported cases of cross-infection from resuscitation.

DRESSINGS AND BANDAGES

The standard First Aid box will contain medium and large wound dressings for the purpose of controlling bleeding and preventing infection. Each dressing is wrapped sterile and should only be used if the wrapping is intact and the shelf life is in date. Smaller and larger dressings may be added to the First Aid box if required.

STERILE DRESSING

TRIANGULAR BANDAGE

The general principles for using wound dressings:
- Wear gloves
- Check for embedded foreign objects
- Use a sterile dressing
- Select a large enough dressing for the wound
- Keep the dressing rolled whilst applying
- Hold dressings by the edges, not the pad
- Place the pad over the wound and bandage firmly but not too tightly by wrapping the long part of the bandage completely around the pad
- Tie off using a reef knot, safety pin or tape
- Check that circulation is not impeded beyond the wound
- Keep a check on the dressing to ensure the bleeding has stopped
- If bleeding persists apply a second dressing on top of the first
- If this does not control the bleeding, remove the two dressings and start again

The only bandages you will find in a standard First Aid box are triangular bandages. These can be used flat or folded into a broad or narrow- fold bandage to help support a limb or to assist in applying pressure over a sterile dressing.

How to turn a triangular bandage into a broad-fold bandage

Point

Base

End

Open triangular bandage

Point

Base

End

First folded edge aligned with base

THE TREATMENT OF MINOR EXTERNAL BLEEDING

Rest
Elevate
Direct pressure

With minor bleeding from cuts and abrasions the emphasis is on keeping the wound clean to control any blood loss.

- Wear disposable gloves
- Examine the injury for any embedded foreign objects
- Clean the wound under fresh running water
- Sit the casualty down. If they feel weak and unsteady, position them on the floor
- Clean the skin around the wound with wet sterile gauze or sterile non-alcoholic wipes
- Elevate the injury to control any blood loss
- Dry the wound with sterile gauze and apply a plaster or sterile dressing
- Advise the casualty to seek medical attention if necessary

DISPOSABLE GLOVES

THE TREATMENT OF MAJOR EXTERNAL BLEEDING

With severe wounds and bleeding the emphasis is on controlling blood loss and treating for shock.

- Wear disposable gloves
- Position the casualty lying down on the floor to help prevent shock
- Examine the injury to establish the extent of the wound and to check for any foreign embedded objects
- Elevate the injured part if injuries allow
- Apply direct pressure over the wound to control blood loss
- Apply a sterile dressing of the appropriate size for the wound
- If bleeding continues through the dressing, apply another one on top
- If bleeding continues through both dressings, remove the two dressings and start again
- Ensure that you have positioned the dressing directly over the wound
- Support the injured part and treat the casualty for shock. Keep them warm and do not let them have anything to eat, drink or smoke
- Call 999/112 for an ambulance and monitor the casualty's condition.

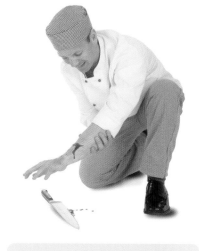

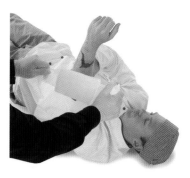

Lying the casualty down on the floor will help prevent shock.

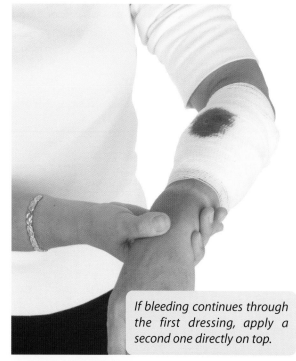

If bleeding continues through the first dressing, apply a second one directly on top.

Support the injured part and treat the casualty for shock. Keep them warm and do not let them have anything to eat, drink or smoke.

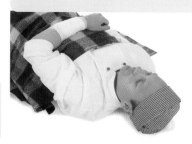

In cases where injuries have caused severe damage to the arm or leg you may find that direct pressure and elevation are insufficient. If the bleeding cannot be controlled, you will have to apply indirect pressure on the artery above the wound.

Indirect pressure should only be used when the bleeding cannot be brought under control by conventional means or when you are unable to apply direct pressure and elevation. This would apply with a casualty who is trapped and where you cannot gain sufficient access to the wound directly.

There are two places where a First Aider can apply indirect pressure:
○ The brachial artery in the arm
○ The femoral artery in the upper leg

Indirect pressure should not be maintained for longer than 10 minutes. After this, release the pressure slowly. If bleeding still persists, apply pressure again whilst waiting for an ambulance. Inform the ambulance crew on the action you have taken and for how long.

WOUNDS WITH EMBEDDED FOREIGN OBJECTS

○ Wear disposable gloves
○ Position the casualty lying down on the floor to help prevent shock
○ Examine the injury to establish the extent of the wound and to check for any embedded foreign objects
○ Elevation of the injured part may be difficult if the object is likely to cause further damage and pain
○ Do not remove the object
○ Apply pressure on either side of the object to control blood loss
○ If the object is large, apply rolled sterile dressings to the wound around the object and bandage firmly in place with a figure of eight method
○ If the object is small, the wound may be covered lightly with a sterile pad before building up around it. Do not apply any pressure directly on top of the object

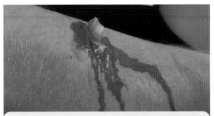

Wound with embedded foreign object (glass).

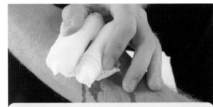

Apply dressings and pressure to either side of the object.

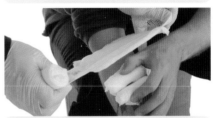

Apply larger dressing.

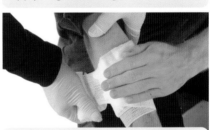

Ask the casualty to assist if able.

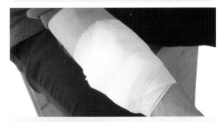

Secure the bandage.

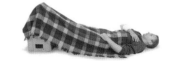

Treat for shock.

THE TREATMENT OF EXTERNAL BLEEDING TO THE SCALP

- ○ Wear disposable gloves
- ○ Position the casualty lying down on the floor. Raise the head and shoulders slightly to reduce blood flow
- ○ Be aware of any fractures to the skull and spine before elevating
- ○ Examine the injury to establish the extent of the wound and to check for any foreign objects
- ○ Apply direct pressure over the wound
- ○ Apply a sterile dressing of the appropriate size for the wound
- ○ Secure the dressing in place with a head bandage
- ○ Call 999/112 for an ambulance and monitor the casualty's condition
- ○ If the casualty becomes unconscious carry out your procedure for Basic Life Support

THE TREATMENT OF EXTERNAL BLEEDING TO THE HAND

- ○ Wear disposable gloves
- ○ Position the casualty lying down on the floor. Elevate the arm to reduce blood flow
- ○ Be aware of any fractures before elevating
- ○ Examine the injury to establish the extent of the wound and to check for any foreign objects
- ○ Apply direct pressure on the wound with an open sterile dressing and encourage the casualty to form a fist
- ○ Position another sterile dressing over the fist and wrap around the entire hand to keep the fist clenched
- ○ Remove any watches or rings before applying pressure
- ○ Keep the injury elevated and obtain medical assistance
- ○ If the hand cannot be clenched because of injury to bones or tendons, treat as per normal external bleeding

THE TREATMENT OF BLEEDING FROM THE EAR

Bleeding from the ear may be as a direct result from external injuries such as a fractured skull, a human bite or a foreign object. There is also the possibility of a ruptured eardrum from a blast injury or an infection. If the blood coming from the ear is mixed with a clear fluid you should suspect a fractured skull.

- ○ Wear disposable gloves
- ○ Position the casualty in a half-sitting position on the floor with the head tilted to the injured side
- ○ Be aware of any fractures to the skull and neck before positioning the casualty
- ○ Examine the ear to establish the extent of the wound and to check for any foreign objects
- ○ Apply a dressing lightly over the ear and secure in place
- ○ Do not plug the ear
- ○ If the casualty becomes unconscious as a result of the injury, carry out your procedures for Basic Life Support and position them in the recovery position with the injured ear nearest the floor

THE TREATMENT OF BLEEDING FROM THE NOSE

Nose bleeds are common and are often caused by hard blowing of the nose during a cold, a foreign object, a punch or a build-up of pressure as a result of stress or nervousness. If the blood coming from the nose is mixed with a clear fluid you should suspect a fractured skull.

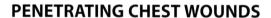

- Wear disposable gloves
- Sit the casualty up and leaning forward
- Check for fractures to the skull and neck before positioning
- Examine the nose to establish the extent of any wound and to check for foreign objects
- Assist them to pinch the soft part of the nose just below the bridge
- Keep this pressure on for about 10 minutes and release slowly
- When the bleeding is under control advise them not to blow their nose for a few hours
- If the bleeding persists, carry out the procedure for a further 10 minutes. If this does not stop the bleeding, continue the procedure and send them to hospital

PENETRATING CHEST WOUNDS

Injuries to the chest can cause fractured ribs and damage to the heart and lungs. When the chest wall is punctured, air will be sucked in through the opening as the casualty breathes in. This will cause pressure to build and the lungs to collapse as the air fills the cavity surrounding the lungs. This can also lead to pressure being exerted on the heart. The injuries may also cause internal bleeding inside the cavity, therefore increasing the pressure.

RECOGNITION
- Signs of shock and hypoxia
- Coughed-up frothy red blood
- A crackling feeling around the site of the wound
- Blood bubbling out of the wound
- The sound of air being sucked into the chest as the casualty breathes in
- One side of the chest being sucked in as the other side expands
- Distressed breathing

TREATMENT
- Immediately call 999/112 for an ambulance and put on your gloves
- Apply direct pressure over the wound
- Position the casualty in a half sitting position or lying down with the head and shoulders raised
- Incline the casualty towards the injured side
- Apply a sterile dressing over the wound
- Apply plastic material such as kitchen film over the dressing and tape in place on three sides. Leave the bottom side open as this will allow air to escape and relieve some of the pressure
- If a foreign object is embedded in the chest, leave it in place
- Maintain the casualty in this position unless they become unconscious
- Place them in the recovery position injured side down

ABDOMINAL WOUNDS

The abdomen lies beneath the ribcage and above the pelvic cavity. There are no bony structures to protect the internal organs. The abdominal cavity is home to the stomach, liver, spleen, intestines, pancreas and kidneys. This cavity is surrounded by numerous layers of muscles apart from the area around the spine and lower ribs. Any injury to this area will result in severe loss of blood both internally and externally.

Abdominal wounds are normally as a result of severe trauma like that seen in road traffic accidents, blast injuries, crush injuries or stabbing. Unlike other wounds where you may only have to treat bleeding. The abdominal wound, if deep, will cause the intestines to protrude through the wound.

RECOGNITION
- A history of abdominal injury
- Bleeding from a wound with the possibility of visible intestines
- Muscle spasms, cramps and severe pain within the abdomen
- Nausea and vomiting
- All the signs and symptoms of shock
- Tenderness and rigidity of the abdominal wall
- Bruising and discolouration

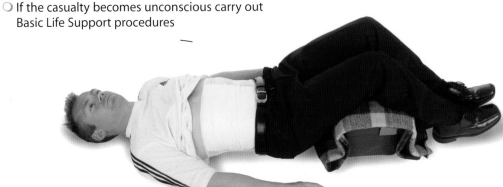

TREATMENT
- Immediately call 999/112 for an ambulance and put on your gloves
- Position the casualty lying down and the knees drawn up
- Apply direct pressure to the wound with a sterile dressing only if nothing is protruding from the wound
- Secure the dressing with a broad-fold triangular bandage for extra support
- If the casualty coughs, apply hand pressure over the dressing to prevent the intestines from errupting out through the wound
- If part of the intestine is protruding do not allow it to become dry
- Before applying a dressing cover the wound with a plastic material such as kitchen film or a wet dressing. Do not touch the intestines or attempt to push them back in
- If the casualty becomes unconscious carry out Basic Life Support procedures

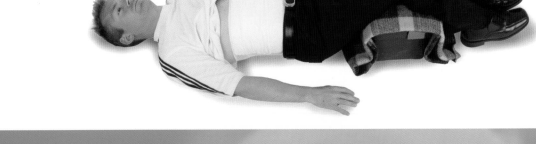

AMPUTATIONS

Amputation of a body part will not only cause a loss of blood and damage to bone, tendons, ligament and muscle, but also shock from pain and losing a body part.

If the amputation is complete you should always attempt to preserve the amputated part as prompt medical attention may save the limb or digit.

RECOGNITION
- Severe bleeding if the amputation was due to blunt trauma *(crushed or torn off)*
- In cases of sharp trauma where the body part has been cleanly cut off, the blood vessels at the site will often constrict to reduce the amount of blood loss
- Severe pain, anxiety and shock

TREATMENT
- Wear gloves
- Control blood loss by means of direct pressure and elevation
- Apply a sterile dressing directly over the wound
- In severe cases, you may have to apply indirect pressure
- Treat the casualty for shock and give them nothing to eat, drink or smoke
- Place the amputated part in a plastic bag or kitchen film
- Wrap a cloth around the plastic
- Place the body part in a bag of ice
- Clearly identify the amputated part and name of the casualty on the bag
- Call 999/112 for an ambulance and monitor their condition

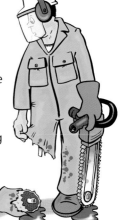

- **Do not** allow the body part to have direct contact with the ice
- **Do not** wash or attempt to clean the body part
- **Do not** wrap in cotton wool

CRUSH INJURIES

When part of the body is crushed, blood cannot circulate freely beyond the crush. The toxins created by the waste products that would normally be carried away in the blood are not allowed to return, causing a build-up below the crush point.

If the object causing the crush is removed suddenly, the build-up of toxins will be too great for the kidneys to filter. This could lead to serious damage or complete kidney failure. This is known as crush syndrome.

TREATMENT
- The First Aider must establish how long the crush has been in place. If it has not been in place for more than 15 minutes, and it is safe to approach the casualty, you can remove the crush
- Treat any wounds and bleeding as normal
- Treat for shock but be aware of injuries to the spine and legs
- If the crush has been in place for longer than 15 minutes leave in place
- Call 999/112 for an ambulance and monitor the casualty
- The release rule of 15 minutes does not apply if the crush is to the head, neck or chest
- Advise the medical personnel of how long the crush has been in place or when it was removed

EYE INJURIES

Eye injuries caused by a blow or foreign objects on or in the eye are painful and distressing. Whatever the cause, it should be remembered that any form of eye injury could have a serious effect on the casualty's sight. This could not only result from the injury but as a result of infection.

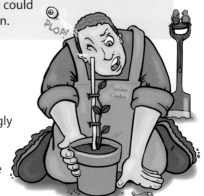

TREATMENT
- Wear gloves
- Position the casualty on the floor with the head and shoulders raised and the head supported
- Examine the eye for foreign objects and treat accordingly See Section 16 for detailed treatment for minor injuries to the eye
- Place a sterile dressing over the eye and secure in place if necessary
- Ask the casualty to keep both eyes still as any movement may cause further damage to the injured eye. Send to hospital calling 999/112 if necessary

INTERNAL BLEEDING

Internal bleeding can be caused by damage to internal organs from a blow, fall or crush. It can also be caused by fractures that have punctured blood vessels, muscle tissue or organs, or as a result of internal rupture.

RECOGNITION
- All the signs and symptoms of shock
- No visible signs of external bleeding on the body
- Pain
- Thirst
- Confusion, restlessness and irritability
- Possible collapse
- Pattern bruising/swelling
- Bleeding from orifices

BLEEDING FROM ORIFICES

BLEEDING FROM THE MOUTH
Injury to the lungs if the blood that is coughed up is bright red and frothy.
Bleeding in the digestive system if the blood is dark red, reddish brown and vomited up.

BLEEDING FROM THE EAR
Injury to the ear or a perforated ear drum if the blood is bright red.
Head injury if the blood is mixed with a clear fluid.

BLEEDING FROM THE ANUS
Injury to the anus or lower bowel if the blood is bright red.
Injury to the upper bowel if the blood is dark red with offensive tarry stools.

BLEEDING IN THE URINARY SYSTEM

Injury or disease in the bladder, kidneys and urethra if the urine has a cloudy appearance with traces of blood and possible clotting.

BLEEDING FROM THE VAGINA

Menstruation, miscarriage, disease or injury to the vagina or womb. The blood may be bright or dark red.

TREATMENT FOR INTERNAL BLEEDING

When treating a casualty for internal bleeding you should also be treating the cause of the injury. If fractures are suspected, it may be difficult to move the casualty into a shock position.

Internal bleeding will cause pressure on various internal organs. Bleeding in the skull will put pressure on the brain and bleeding in the abdomen will put pressure on the diaphragm and interfere with normal breathing.

You will need to treat the casualty for shock but if the bleeding is in the chest or abdominal cavity laying them down with the legs raised will increase the pressure on the internal organs and make breathing difficult. Position the casualty in a semi-seated position with the knees bent and supported underneath.

○ Treat the casualty for shock

○ Call 999/112 for an ambulance

○ Monitor the casualty's condition

○ Calm and reassure them

○ If the casualty becomes unconscious, carry out your procedures for Basic Life Support

○ When placing them in the recovery position, lay them with the injured side down

○ In treating bleeding from the vagina or anus, you will be dealing with a sensitive area of the body which is likely to cause much embarrassment. Try to gain their confidence and ask for assistance from another person, preferably a female if the casualty is a female

○ If bleeding is present at the vagina or the anus, ask the casualty to hold a large sterile dressing in place

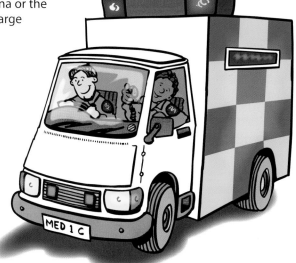

FIRST AID at work

SECTION SUMMARY

THE MAIN TYPES OF WOUND ARE:
- Incision
- Laceration
- Contusion
- Abrasion
- Puncture
- Velocity injury

THE TYPES OF BLEEDING ARE:
- Arterial
- Venous
- Capillary

HOW CAN YOU HELP TO PREVENT CROSS-INFECTION WHEN TREATING MINOR BLEEDING?
- Wash your hands
- Wear gloves
- Do not cough, talk or breathe directly over a wound
- Clean the wound
- Use sterile dressings
- Dispose of soiled dressings correctly

HOW MANY DRESSINGS SHOULD YOU APPLY TO A WOUND?
- Two, and if the bleeding continues, remove them and start again

HOW SHOULD YOU TREAT A WOUND WITH AN EMBEDDED FOREIGN OBJECT?
- Leave the object in place and dress around it. Secure in place with another dressing

HOW SHOULD YOU TREAT MAJOR BLEEDING?
- Wear gloves
- Position the casualty
- Expose and examine the wound
- Elevate the injured part
- Apply direct pressure
- Apply a sterile dressing
- Treat for shock
- Check that circulation is not interrupted

HOW WOULD YOU RECOGNISE INTERNAL BLEEDING?
- Swelling
- Bruising
- Pain
- Discomfort
- Bleeding from orifices
- Signs and symptoms of shock

HOW SHOULD YOU TREAT A WOUND TO THE EYE?

- ○ Lay the casualty down
- ○ Examine the injury
- ○ Cover with a sterile dressing
- ○ Ask the casualty to remain calm and still
- ○ Encourage the casualty not to move the other eye

HOW SHOULD YOU TREAT AN AMPUTATION?

- ○ Treat as for major bleeding
- ○ Place the amputated part in a plastic bag
- ○ Cover with a cloth
- ○ Place this in a bag or on a bed of ice

HOW SHOULD YOU TREAT A CRUSH INJURY?

- ○ Only remove the crushing object if it has been in place for less than 15 minutes or if breathing is compromised

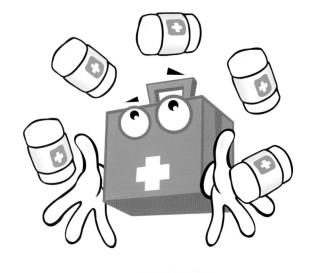

BITES AND STINGS

Although many stings and bites are painful, most are not usually serious. Human bites are very painful and may cause considerable blood loss and infection. Animal bites, for example from cats and dogs, are puncture wounds that can carry infection deep inside the body. Insect bites and stings can be an irritation and are sometimes painful. There is also a risk of localised swelling and anaphylactic shock. Any bite or sting in the mouth or throat can lead to swelling and obstruction of the airway.

TREATMENT

The general treatment for all types of bites and stings:
- Ensure safety
- Wear gloves
- Keep the casualty still to limit the effects of any venom
- Control any bleeding
- Minimize the risk of infection by keeping the area covered and clean
- Monitor the airway and breathing
- Call medical attention if necessary
- Do not remove any stings with tweezers. Try to brush them off with a blunt edge.

There are specific treatments relating to the cause when treating bites and stings from marine creatures or snakes. Although the reactions are generally mild, the young and elderly can experience greater difficulties.

Jelly fish and sea anemones have stinging cells that stick to the skin. These contain venom and although relatively harmless in the UK, this venom can cause swelling and anaphylactic reactions.

- Brush off the cells with powdered chalk or pour vinegar over the affected area to neutralize the cells
- Keep the casualty still to limit the effects of any venom and apply a cold pack to reduce any swelling
- Monitor the airway and breathing
- Send to hospital or call 999/112 if necessary

Creatures such as weaver fish and sea urchins have spines containing venom as a defence against attack. These spines penetrate the skin and can be difficult to remove. Venom from these creatures can produce massive swelling. This can obstruct circulation, cause infection and on occasions can cause paralysis and cardiac arrest.

- Sit the casualty down and immerse the foot or hand in hot water. This helps to draw the venom back towards the injury site
- Calm and reassure the casualty as they will be in considerable pain
- Send to hospital or call 999/112 for an ambulance
- The spines should only be removed at the hospital
- Keep the injured area clean to minimize the risk of infection

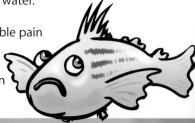

Snake bites in the UK are rare and not usually fatal unless the snake has been imported. These can cause varying reactions such as pain, swelling, vomiting, sweating, disturbed vision, weakness and breathing difficulties.

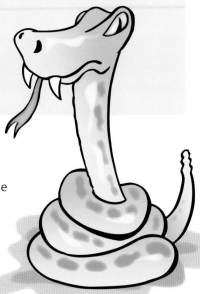

○ Position the casualty on the floor in a seated position to keep them still
○ Clean the bite area
○ Bandage the injured part tightly with a crepe bandage if available, in order to reduce the circulation and the flow of venom. Do not over tighten and stop the circulation altogether
○ Immobilize the affected part and keep it below the level of the heart
○ Calm and reassure the casualty
○ If the casualty becomes weak or unconscious, place them in the recovery position on the injured side
○ Monitor the casualty's airway and breathing. Be prepared to carry out the procedures for Basic Life Support.

DISORDERS OF CONSCIOUSNESS

Our nervous system is extremely complex, but for the purpose of First Aid we only need an understanding of the basics. The nervous system contains billions of nerve cells called neurons. Between the brain and the skull there is a clear fluid called cerebrospinal fluid that acts as a shock absorber for the brain and carries oxygen and nutrients. The central nervous system is composed of the brain and spinal cord. In general the brain acts upon the stimuli it receives from the nerves but some actions such as reflex actions, are controlled by the spinal cord. The peripheral or voluntary nervous system is made up of two sets of nerves. The cranial nerves stem from the underside of the brain and the spinal nerves which emerge from the spinal cord extend throughout the vertebral column. These nerves relay information from and to the central nervous system via the spinal cord for motor and sensory impulses. The autonomic nervous system is made up of some cranial nerves and some spinal nerves, thus being an integral part of the peripheral nervous system. This system controls the vital functions of the body such as breathing, circulation, digestion, blinking and body temperature.

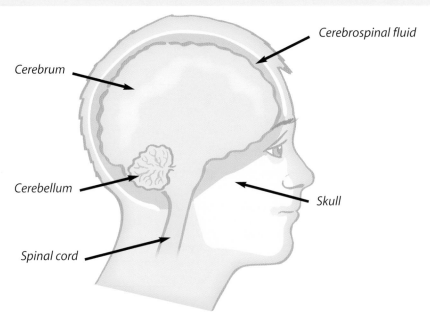

This section covers medical conditions and injuries that affect the brain and the nervous system such as:

Injury to the head, brain or spinal cord
○ Stroke
○ Diabetes
○ Epilepsy

There are numerous conditions that will lead to unconsciousness such as poisons, hypothermia and heatstroke. For ease of reference and to avoid confusion, these conditions are covered in separate sections.

HEAD INJURIES

With minor blows or falls the skull is usually able to provide adequate protection for the brain. When the injury is of a more serious nature the skull could fracture and lead to damage to the brain. All injuries to the head should be treated as serious as they are potentially dangerous. Medical assistance should be obtained in all cases.

CONCUSSION

Concussion can best be described as a shaking of the brain leading to a brief loss of consciousness. This is often caused by a direct force such as a blow to the head or an indirect force as with whiplash in a car accident.

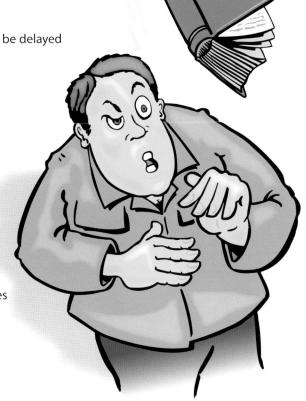

RECOGNITION
- Brief loss of consciousness which may be delayed
- Dizziness and mild headache
- Nausea
- Loss of memory
- Disturbed vision
- Pale, cold and clammy skin

TREATMENT
- Sit the conscious casualty down or place in the recovery position if they are weak and unsteady
- If unconscious and breathing, place them in the recovery position
- Monitor the airway, breathing and response levels
- Seek medical assistance
- If unconscious for more than 3 minutes dial 999/112 for an ambulance
- Do not let the casualty drive or play any sports until seen by a doctor

CEREBRAL COMPRESSION

Cerebral compression is a very serious condition and needs urgent medical attention. Pressure is exerted on the brain from bleeding inside the skull, the build up of blood on the surface of the brain, a skull fracture or even infection. The most common cause of cerebral compression is a head injury, but the signs and symptoms may not always be immediately recognisable. In some cases the condition can take a number of days to develop.

RECOGNITION

- Evidence of a head injury
- Intense headache
- Slow and noisy breathing
- Slow and strong pulse
- Unequal pupils
- High temperature
- Flushed appearance
- Muscle twitching on one side of the body
- Drowsiness and change in personality
- Paralysis and weakness of the limbs
- Skull fracture could lead to fluid escaping from the ears and nose

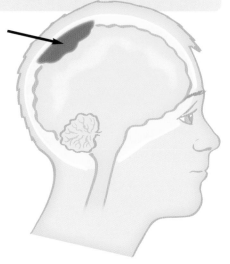

Build up of blood

TREATMENT

- If conscious, lay the casualty down and raise the head and shoulders
- Monitor the airway, breathing and response levels
- Loosen tight clothing to make the casualty comfortable. Keep them warm
- Reassure
- Dial 999/112 for an ambulance
- If unconscious and breathing, leave the casualty in the position found and maintain their airway as there may be damage to the neck
- Monitor the casualty's airway and breathing. Be prepared to carry out the procedures for Basic Life Support
- Do not give the casualty anything to eat, drink or smoke

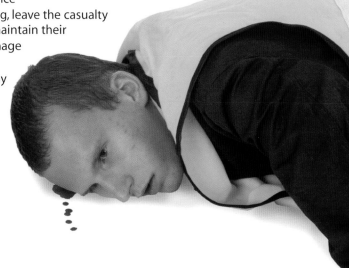

FRACTURED SKULL

Fractures to the skull mainly occur in two places. The dome or vault of the skull can be fractured by a heavy blow leading to a depressed fracture. An indirect force such as landing awkwardly from a fall or receiving a blow to the jaw could fracture the base of the skull.

If the skull is fractured, there is a strong indication of injury to the spine, so steps should be taken not to move the casualty unless absolutely necessary.

There may be a wound with a depressed fracture that will allow infection inside the skull if left untreated. You may also see evidence of concussion and compression.

RECOGNITION

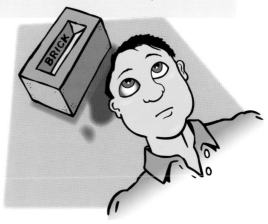

- Evidence of head injury and unconsciousness
- A wound, bruise or depression in the skull
- Deterioration in response levels
- Fluids from the ears and nose
- Blood in the whites of the eyes
- Distortion of the head and face
- Associated spinal injury

TREATMENT

- Dial 999/112 for an ambulance
- Control any bleeding and fluid loss
- If you suspect spinal injury, do not move the casualty
- If unconscious and breathing, leave the casualty in the position found and maintain their airway as there may be damage to the neck
- If you are unable to maintain the airway, turn them into the recovery position by means of the log roll
- If you are able to move them, lay them down and raise the head and shoulders.
- Monitor the casualty's airway and breathing. Be prepared to carry out the procedures for Basic Life Support
- If rescue breaths are needed, open the airway with the normal head-tilt-chin lift.

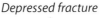

Depressed fracture

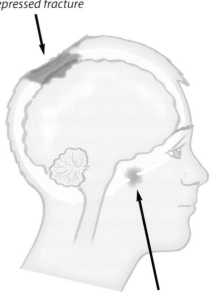

Base of skull fracture

Section 14

STROKE

A stroke is a sudden attack that is primarily caused by an interruption or reduction of the blood supply to the brain. This occurs when the flow of blood is prevented from reaching the brain by a blood clot or by a rupture of an artery supplying the brain. The severity of the attack can vary from a weakness and partial paralysis of the face and limbs, to a loss in control of normal bodily functions, paralysis and death.

RECOGNITION
- Sudden severe headache
- Confused and emotional
- Sudden or gradual loss of consciousness
- Drunken appearance
- Paralysis down one side of the body, unequal pupils, dribbling
- Paralysis of the facial muscles on one side
- Loss of bladder and bowel control

TREATMENT
- If conscious, lay the casualty down and raise the head and shoulders. Turn their head to one side and place a cloth or dressing on the shoulder for any dribbling
- Monitor the airway, breathing and response levels
- Loosen tight clothing to make the casualty comfortable
- Reassure and dial 999/112 for an ambulance
- If unconscious, place the casualty in the recovery position injured side down. Be prepared to carry out your procedure for Basic Life Support

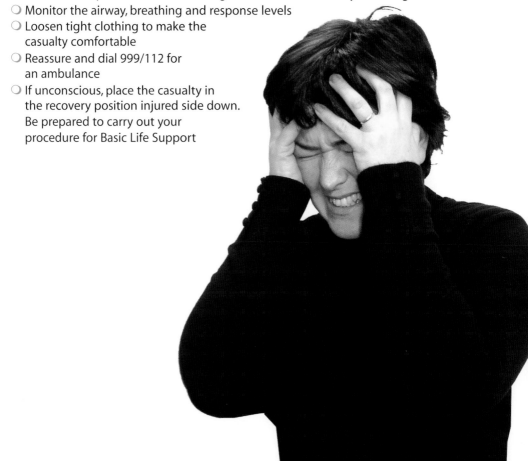

EPILEPSY

There are more than forty different types of epilepsy. For the First Aider we look at them as minor and major seizures.

Epilepsy is a disorder of brain function that can be brought on by head injuries, emotional upset, anxiety, a reaction to certain foods, changes in body temperature, vibration and tiredness.

Minor seizures or absence seizures are a brief loss of consciousness sometimes only lasting for a few seconds. Convulsive movements usually accompany major seizures.

MINOR EPILEPSY RECOGNITION
- Sudden absence
- Staring blankly ahead
- Slight twitching of the face, lips, eyes and limbs
- Chewing and lip smacking
- Plucking at clothing
- Noises

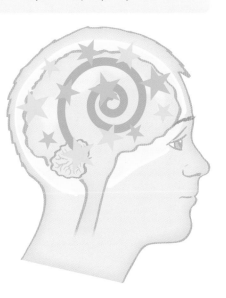

MINOR EPILEPSY TREATMENT
- Make the casualty safe. Sit them down, calm and reassure them
- Monitor and discuss the condition with the casualty
- Establish a history of the condition and if medication is being taken
- Refer to a doctor if necessary

MAJOR EPILEPSY RECOGNITION
- A warning period. The casualty has strange sensations
- The casualty becomes rigid and often cries out
- Sudden collapse and becomes unconscious (tonic phase)
- Cyanosis may be present and breathing may cease
- Convulsive movement which can be violent (clonic phase)
- Loss of bladder or bowel control
- Clenched jaw and congestion of the face

MAJOR EPILEPSY TREATMENT
- Make the area safe and clear the area around the casualty
- Do not restrain the casualty but make them comfortable
- Place padding under their head to stop any injury
- Do not put anything in their mouth
- Loosen tight restrictive clothing
- Record the duration of the seizure
- Dial 999/112 if the seizure lasts for more than five minutes, if the casualty has multiple seizures, if it is their first seizure, if they injure themselves or if the seizure took place in water (possible secondary drowning)
- Place in the recovery position and monitor until they have recovered

DIABETES

Diabetes Mellitus is a medical condition caused by the failure of the body to regulate the blood sugar levels. Blood sugar levels are regulated by insulin produced in the pancreas.

Low levels of insulin and high sugar intake increase the blood sugar that leads to HYPERglycaemia (high blood sugar). This usually develops over a number of days. This can be controlled with diet, insulin injections or tablets. Too much insulin or too little sugar can cause HYPOglycaemia.

Hyperglycaemia and Hypoglycaemia can be recognised as follows:

	HYPERglycaemia	HYPOglycaemia
Amount of insulin used	Not enough	Too much
Deterioration	Gradual	Very quick
Hunger	Absent	Present
Vomiting	Common	Uncommon
Thirst	Present	Absent
Breath odour	Fruity/sweet	Normal
Pulse	Rapid and weak	Rapid
Breathing	Rapid	Normal
Skin	Dry and warm	Pale, cold and sweaty
Seizures	Uncommon	Common
Consciousness	Drowsy	Rapid loss

TREATMENT OF HYPERGLYCAEMIA
- Call for an ambulance 999/112
- If the casualty becomes unconscious place them in the recovery position
- Monitor their breathing and response levels

TREATMENT OF HYPOGLYCAEMIA
- Sit the casualty down
- Give them a sugary drink
- If this is effective give them more
- Follow this with sweet food
- Monitor and reassure them
- If the sugary drink has no effect dial 999/112
- If they become unconscious, put the casualty in the recovery position and monitor

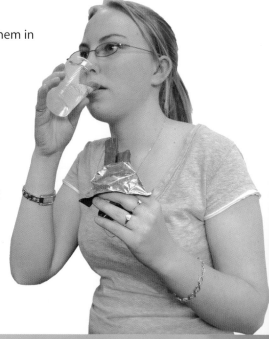

SECTION SUMMARY

WHAT ARE SOME OF THE MAIN CAUSES OF UNCONSCIOUSNESS?
- Fainting
- Shock
- Stroke
- Head injury
- Asphyxia
- Epilepsy
- Diabetes
- Poisoning (See section 19)
- Heart attack

WHAT IS CONCUSSION?
- A shaking of the brain leading to a brief loss of consciousness

WHAT IS CEREBRAL COMPRESSION?
- A bleed or a blood clot on the surface of the brain

HOW SHOULD YOU TREAT COMPRESSION?
- If you do not suspect spinal injury lay the casualty down with the head and shoulders raised
- Treat any wounds to the head
- Keep the casualty warm and reassured
- Call for an ambulance

WHAT COULD CAUSE A FRACTURED SKULL?
- A direct or an indirect force to the head

WHY SHOULD YOU LEAVE A CONSCIOUS BREATHING CASUALTY WITH A FRACTURED SKULL IN THE POSITION FOUND?
- In case of damage to the spine

WHAT IS EPILEPSY?
- A disorder of normal brain functions caused by an electrical disturbance

HOW SHOULD YOU TREAT A CASUALTY SUFFERING FROM A STROKE?
- Lay the casualty down
- Slightly raise the head and shoulders
- Keep them warm
- Constantly monitor any changes in their condition
- Calm and reassure them
- Call for an ambulance
- Be prepared to resuscitate

WHAT IS DIABETES?
- A failure of the body to regulate the blood sugar levels

WHAT IS THE INITIAL TREATMENT FOR A CASUALTY WITH HYPOGLYCAEMIA?
- Sit the casualty down and give them a sugary drink

Section 15

FOREIGN OBJECTS

Any object, large or small, that finds its way into the body either through a wound in the skin or via one of the body's orifices is called a foreign object. Although the initial injury may be minor, foreign objects in the eye, nose, mouth and ear can lead to complications and infection.

The aim in dealing with any foreign object is to decide if it is safe to remove it or to refer the casualty to hospital.

Any object that is embedded must be left in place and protected.

Objects such as splinters, glass or pieces of grit in the skin must not be removed with tweezers or sharp instruments. If the object will not brush off with the finger or a blunt edge, cover with a sterile dressing and seek medical attention.

FOREIGN OBJECT IN THE NOSE
○ Objects pushed up the nose may cause blockages or infection
○ Keep the casualty calm and reassure
○ Get the casualty to breathe through the mouth
○ Do not attempt to remove the object
○ Send the casualty to hospital

FOREIGN OBJECT IN THE EAR
○ This may cause temporary deafness or it may damage the eardrum
○ Do not attempt to remove the object. You may cause serious injury or push the object further inside
○ Cover with a sterile dressing
○ Send the casualty to hospital
○ For insects in the ear you should flood the ear with tepid water so that the insect floats out. If this is unsuccessful send the casualty to hospital

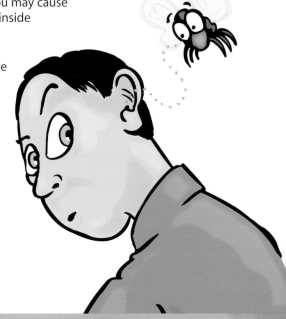

FOREIGN OBJECT IN THE EYE

- ○ Your aim is to prevent injury and infection to the eye
- ○ Advise the casualty not to rub the eye
- ○ Separate the eyelids with the finger and thumb
- ○ If you can see a foreign object on the white of the eye wash it out with clean water or sterile eyewash
- ○ Do not touch anything that is embedded in the eye as you may scratch the surface.
- ○ Cover and send to hospital
- ○ Do not poke anything into the eye to remove an object
- ○ Eyes are extremely vulnerable to infection. Only use sterile eye dressings to cover the eye

Do not touch anything that is embedded in the eye. Your aim is to flush the object from the eye, using clean water or sterile eyewash.

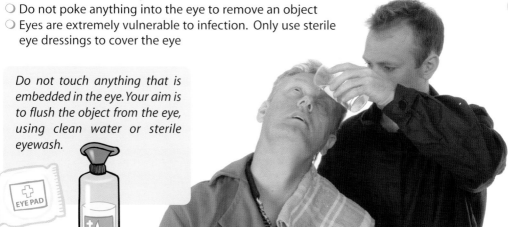

SWALLOWED FOREIGN OBJECTS

- ○ Any object that is swallowed can cause complications to the digestive system. Objects such as fish bones can become stuck in the airway and cause inflammation
- ○ For all swallowed objects send the casualty to hospital
- ○ Do not give the casualty anything to eat or drink as an anaesthetic may have to be administered
- ○ If the object has become lodged in the airway you may have to treat for choking

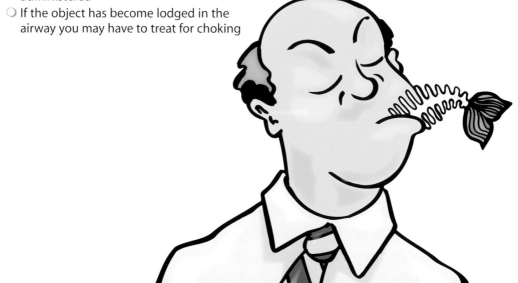

BURNS AND SCALDS

Contact with any source of heat, radiation, electricity, chemical or freezing surface will cause a burn or scald. Burns are among the most serious and painful of all injuries causing damage to the skin, underlying tissue and vital organs. Although a burn may be the most obvious injury you should always perform a complete assessment to determine if there are other serious injuries.

CAUSES OF BURNS

DRY BURNS
○ Hot surfaces
○ Fire
○ Friction

SCALDS
○ Hot liquids
○ Hot fat or oil
○ Steam

ELECTRICAL BURNS
○ Domestic low voltage appliances
○ Lightning
○ High voltage
○ Cables

RADIATION
○ Sunburn
○ Ultraviolet lamps
○ Overexposure to X-ray

CHEMICAL BURNS
○ Acids and alkalis
○ Domestic cleaning products
○ Industrial chemicals

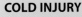

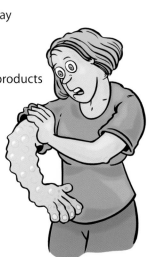

COLD INJURY
○ Freezing temperatures
○ Foreign objects
○ Refrigerants

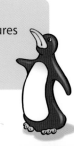

THE DEPTH OF BURNS

SUPERFICIAL BURN
This burn affects the outer layer of the skin causing redness, swelling, tenderness and discomfort such as burning your finger on an iron or sunburn.

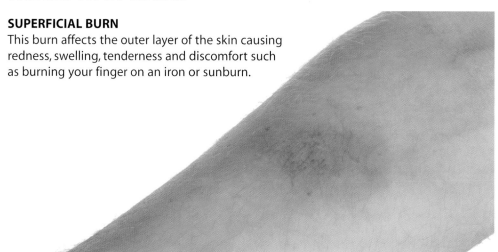

PARTIAL THICKNESS BURN
The outer layer of the skin known as the epidermis has been burnt through causing the skin to become red, raw and swollen with blisters.

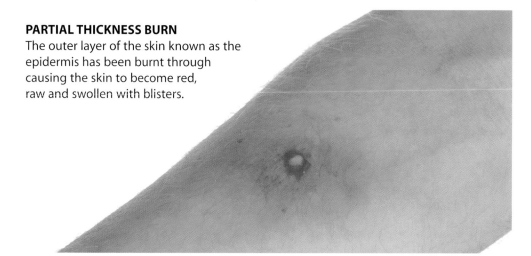

FULL THICKNESS BURN
The two layers of the skin, the epidermis and dermis, are burnt through causing damage to the underlying tissue, nerves and blood vessels. The skin will be charred and waxy with fatty deposits on the surface.

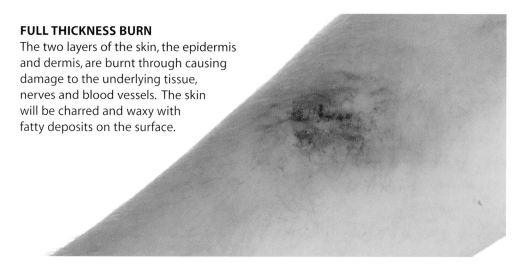

FIRST AID at work

ASSESSING AND TREATING A BURN

When assessing the burnt area the First Aider should consider the following factors, as these will play a large part in the treatment and the recovery of the casualty:

○ Any dangers to yourself, the casualty and any bystanders
○ The age and general condition of the casualty as the degree of shock will increase with the severity of the burn
○ The cause of the burn as there may be more than one burnt area
○ The depth of the burn
○ The extent of the burn will determine if the casualty needs to go to hospital
○ Burns that completely encompass a limb will cause increased swelling and pain
○ Burns to the head and face may cause swelling of the airway and brain
○ Electrical burns will cause damage to underlying tissue and organs

BURNS THAT REQUIRE IMMEDIATE HOSPITAL TREATMENT
○ All burns if the casualty is a child or baby
○ All full thickness burns
○ All burns involving the feet, hands, face or genital area
○ All burns that extend around a limb
○ All partial thickness burns larger than 1% of the casualty's body surface
○ All superficial burns larger than 5% of the casualty's body surface
○ Burns with a mixed pattern of depth
○ If you are unsure about the extent or severity of the burn 1% of the body surface is approximately the size of the casualty's palm

THE TREATMENT OF BURNS AND SCALDS

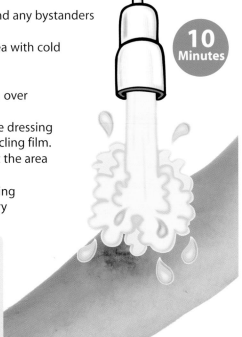

10 Minutes

○ Ensure the safety of yourself, the casualty and any bystanders
○ Wear disposable gloves
○ Reduce the heat by saturating the burnt area with cold water for a minimum of 10 minutes
○ Remove any jewellery or watches
○ Treat for shock as any partial thickness burn over 9% will lead to shock
○ Cover the burnt area with a non-fluffy sterile dressing (burns dressing) or plastic material, such as cling film. Do not wrap too tightly as this will constrict the area if there is swelling
○ Monitor the casualty's response and breathing throughout and send to hospital if necessary

DO NOT:
○ Burst blisters
○ Apply any creams or ointments
○ Remove clothing that is stuck to the skin
○ Apply adhesive dressings
○ Touch the burnt area

TREATING SPECIFIC BURNS

BURNS TO THE AIRWAY
There may be breathing difficulties, soot around the mouth and nose, burnt lips and difficulty in talking.
- ○ Loosen tight clothing
- ○ Remove to the fresh air if possible
- ○ Place the casualty in a seated position
- ○ Monitor the airway and breathing
- ○ Dial 999/112 for an ambulance
- ○ Be prepared to carry out your procedures for Basic Life Support
- ○ Burns to the face and head should be cooled with water but left exposed. Sit the casualty up to reduce swelling

ELECTRICAL BURNS
These may be from the domestic supply, overhead power cables, railway lines or lightning. There may be entry and exit burns on the skin with internal burns following the path of exit. Electric shock may cause cardiac arrest so be prepared to carry out your procedures for Basic Life Support.

WARNING! HIGH VOLTAGE

After ensuring safety, treat as per normal burns and remove to hospital.

If high voltage is involved, call 999/112. Do not approach the casualty until you are officially informed that the power supply has been turned off. Keep a minimum distance of 18 metres from the area.

CHEMICAL BURNS
A First Aider at work should already have an understanding of the chemicals that are used in their own workplace. These may range from irritants to those that will absorb through the skin and cause internal complications.

Although the basic treatment for chemical burns is with cold running water, the First Aider should observe the COSHH assessment of their workplace and be aware of any specific treatments.

- ○ Ensure the area is safe and chemicals have been removed
- ○ Ventilate the area and flood the affected part with cold water for a minimum of 20 minutes
- ○ Remove any contaminated clothing and treat as per normal burns
- ○ Call 999/112 for an ambulance and the Fire Brigade
- ○ If the casualty becomes unconscious, carry out your procedures for Basic Life Support, but be aware that chemicals may have been inhaled

CHEMICAL BURNS TO THE EYE

- Treat as per chemical burns but wash the chemical from the eyes with fresh running water for a minimum of 10 minutes
- Do not let the chemical run into the other eye
- Protect the casualty from any contamination when irrigating
- Cover the eye with a sterile dressing and send to hospital

FLASH BURNS TO THE EYE

Caused by exposure to ultraviolet light or welding equipment

- Redness and pain within the eye
- Gritty feeling in the eye
- Watering of the eye
- Reassure the casualty. Cover the eye with a sterile pad and send to hospital

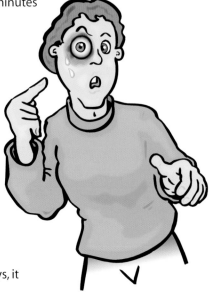

SUNBURN

If this has been caused by overexposure to the sun's rays, it can lead to further complications – heatstroke

- Remove the casualty to a cool place
- Ask them to remove any outer clothing if appropriate and sponge the affected area with cool water for 10 minutes
- If blistering is present, send them to hospital

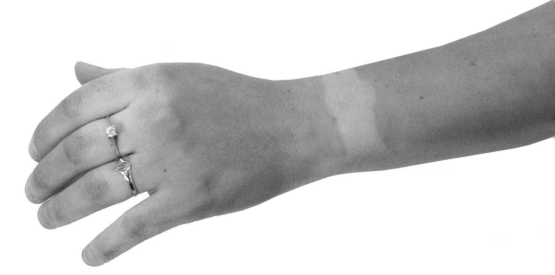

SECTION SUMMARY

WHAT ARE THE MAIN CAUSES OF BURNS?

DRY BURNS
- Fire
- Hot surfaces
- Electrical
- Friction

COLD BURNS
- Freezing temperatures
- Frozen surfaces
- Refrigerants
- Certain gases

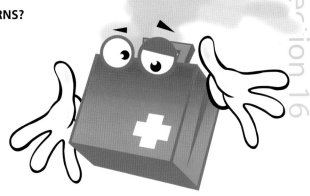

WET BURNS
- Steam
- Hot liquids
- Oils

RADIATION
- Sunburn
- Ultraviolet light

CHEMICALS
- Industrial or household products

HOW SHOULD YOU TREAT A NON-CHEMICAL BURN?
- Cool the burn under running cold water for a minimum of 10 minutes
- Remove any jewellery in case of swelling
- Cover with a sterile, non-fluffy dressing
- Treat for shock
- Call for an ambulance

WHEN SHOULD YOU SEND SOMEONE TO HOSPITAL FOR BURNS?
- When superficial burns are greater than 5%
- When partial thickness burns are greater than 1%
- All full thickness burns

HOW DO YOU CALCULATE THE PERCENTAGE OF BURNS?
- The palm of the hand is equivalent to 1%

WHY SHOULD YOU NEVER BREAK BLISTERS ON A BURN?
- This increases the risk of infection and shock caused by loss of bodily fluid in severe cases

HOW SHOULD YOU TREAT A CHEMICAL BURN?
- ○ Flood the affected area with cold running water for a minimum of 20 minutes
- ○ Remove contaminated clothing if it is not stuck to the skin
- ○ Treat for shock
- ○ Call for an ambulance
- ○ Be aware that certain chemicals require specialist treatment

WHEN TREATING ELECTRICAL BURNS WHAT SHOULD YOU BE LOOKING FOR?
- ○ An entry and exit burn

WHAT IS THE MAIN DANGER OF BURNS TO THE FACE AND NECK?
- ○ Swelling of the airway and smoke inhalation

HOW SHOULD YOU TREAT BURNS TO THE EYES?
- ○ Run cold water over the eye for a minimum of 10 minutes
- ○ Cover with a sterile dressing
- ○ Call for an ambulance

IF THERE HAS BEEN DAMAGE TO HIGH VOLTAGE CABLES WHAT SHOULD YOU DO?
- ○ You should keep a minimum distance of 18 metres from the source

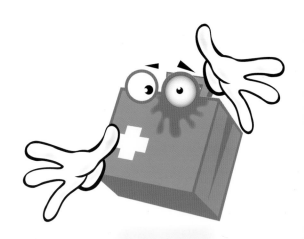

BONE AND MUSCLE INJURY

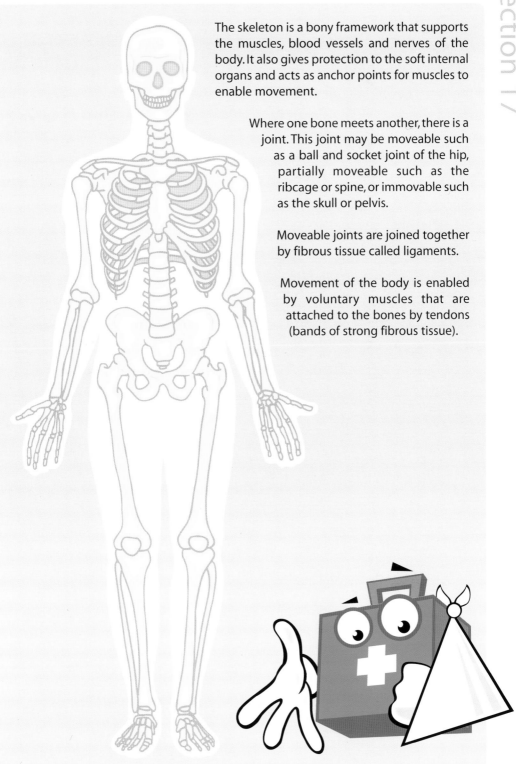

The skeleton is a bony framework that supports the muscles, blood vessels and nerves of the body. It also gives protection to the soft internal organs and acts as anchor points for muscles to enable movement.

Where one bone meets another, there is a joint. This joint may be moveable such as a ball and socket joint of the hip, partially moveable such as the ribcage or spine, or immovable such as the skull or pelvis.

Moveable joints are joined together by fibrous tissue called ligaments.

Movement of the body is enabled by voluntary muscles that are attached to the bones by tendons (bands of strong fibrous tissue).

In this section we will look at injuries to the main structure of the body:

FRACTURE
A crack, chip or break in the bone

DISLOCATION
When two halves of a joint are separated

SPRAIN
A tearing injury to the ligaments surrounding a joint

STRAIN
A tearing injury to muscles and tendons

FRACTURES

There are numerous types of fractures, but in First Aid we only need to look at three main types:

○ A closed fracture is where the broken bone does not puncture the skin
○ An open fracture is where the broken bone has punctured the skin creating a wound and possible infection
○ A complicated fracture can be either closed or open and will involve injury to another part of the body

A closed fracture (left) and an open fracture (right)

CAUSES OF FRACTURES

The following generally cause fractures:

DIRECT FORCE
e.g. slipping on a wet surface and landing on your back or being struck with a blunt object

INDIRECT FORCE
e.g. landing heavily or awkwardly from a fall or jump could cause bones to break in the foot. This would be a direct force but bones in the leg, pelvis, spine and skull could also be fractured as a result of the impact and transference of force.

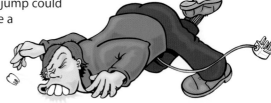

RECOGNITION
- Pain at the site of the injury
- Swelling, deformity and bruising
- A wound with an open fracture
- Irregularity and abnormal appearance
- Lack of movement and power
- Shock
- It would be obvious with an open fracture that a bone is broken but with closed fractures it may not be evident. The only way that a fracture can be correctly diagnosed is by X-ray.

THE TREATMENT OF CLOSED FRACTURES

- Check for dangers to yourself, the casualty and any bystanders
- Assess the situation and look for history of the incident
- Establish that the casualty is responsive and breathing. Carry out your procedures for Basic Life Support if necessary
- Immobilize the injured part to stop any movement
- Support the injured part
- Leave the casualty in the position found unless they can move the injured part to a more comfortable position
- Treat for shock as dictated by the casualty's movements
- Calm and reassure. Call 999/112 for an ambulance and monitor
- In some cases you may be able to take the casualty to hospital. Never take a casualty to hospital on your own as their condition could deteriorate whilst you are driving. The other thing to consider is, does your insurance cover you for the transportation of casualties if you were to have an accident en-route?

THE TREATMENT OF OPEN FRACTURES

- Treat as for a closed fracture
- Control any bleeding and make sure you wear gloves
- Apply sterile dressings around the protruding bone to stop any movement and to minimize the risk of infection
- Do not apply any pressure directly on the wound
- Support and immobilize the injured part in the position found
- Treat for shock
- Call 999/112 for an ambulance

THE TREATMENT OF COMPLICATED FRACTURES

Treat as for a closed or open fracture. Check the casualty for further injury or complications such as a fractured rib penetrating the lung, and treat accordingly.

Effective immobilization sometimes requires the injured part to be secured to an injured body part with bandages and slings. This should only be carried out if an ambulance is not readily available, or if you need to move the casualty to a safer place.

FIRST AID at work

THE TREATMENT OF SPECIFIC FRACTURES

FRACTURES OF THE FACE AND JAW

The treatment of a casualty with facial and jaw fractures is minimal but the First Aider should be aware of possible complications.

A blow to the jaw could also fracture the skull and cause serious breathing difficulties.
○ Carry out your normal checks for response, airway and breathing
○ If the casualty is unconscious and breathing, place them in the recovery position, injured side down, and monitor any changes
○ Be prepared to carry out your procedures for Basic Life Support
○ If the casualty is conscious, place them in a half-sitting position with the head tilted forwards and towards the injured side
○ Provide a sterile dressing or bandage and encourage the casualty to support the jaw with their hands. The dressing will mop up any blood or saliva
○ If a fractured skull is suspected, treat accordingly and monitor

FRACTURED COLLARBONE

A fractured collarbone will require supporting, as the injury and weight of the arm will affect the shoulder joint. The casualty will normally be supporting the arm of the injured side in the most comfortable position.
○ Place the casualty in a seated position
○ Provide a rolled-up blanket or clothing to support the arm of the injured side in the position that the casualty feels most comfortable with
○ Check the pulse at the wrist to ensure that circulation in the arm is present
○ Remove the casualty to hospital if it is safe to do so or call for an ambulance
○ If the ambulance is delayed and providing the casualty will allow you, support the arm of the injured side with an elevated sling and a broad-fold bandage to secure the arm to the body
○ Prompt medical attention is needed, as this type of fracture can damage blood vessels and nerves in the shoulder area

FRACTURED UPPER ARM

As with a fracture to the collarbone any fracture to the upper arm can affect the shoulder joint and cause complications with major blood vessels and nerves.
○ Place the casualty in a seated position
○ Provide a rolled-up blanket or clothing to support the injured arm in the position the casualty feels most comfortable with
○ Check the pulse at the wrist to ensure circulation is present in the arm
○ Remove the casualty to hospital if it is safe to do so or call for an ambulance
○ If the ambulance is delayed and the casualty will allow you, place padding under the arm and support with an arm sling

FRACTURED ELBOW

Depending on the cause of the injury to the elbow, the arm could be straight or bent. The arm must be immobilized in the position found, as any movement will cause serious damage to the major nerves and blood vessels surrounding the elbow joint.
○ Lay the casualty down, as this provides greater support for the injury
○ Place padding between the arm and the body
○ Padding should also be placed in and around any hollows of the body
○ Check the pulse at the wrist to ensure that circulation is present in the arm
○ Make the casualty comfortable and keep them warm
○ Call 999/112 for an ambulance and reassure the casualty

FRACTURED FOREARM AND WRIST

These fractures are common and usually occur when a person falls onto an outstretched arm.

- ◯ Sit the casualty down
- ◯ Place padding under the arm and on the lap to provide support in the position the casualty finds most comfortable
- ◯ Call for an ambulance if the casualty cannot be transported
- ◯ If you do move them and the casualty will allow, immobilize the arm in an arm sling with padding between the arm and the sling

SUPPORT SLING

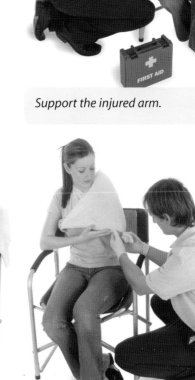

Support the injured arm.

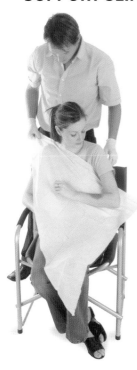

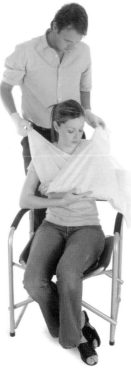

Place a triangular bandage with its base parallel to the casualty's body.

Bring the lower end of the bandage up to meet the upper end at the shoulder. Secure with a reef knot.

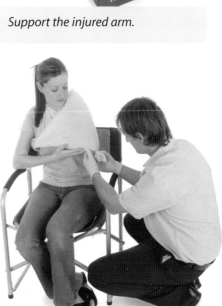

Use a safety pin to secure at elbow or twist bandage and tuck into sling at the back of the arm.

With the arm safely supported in a sling, you can transport the casualty.

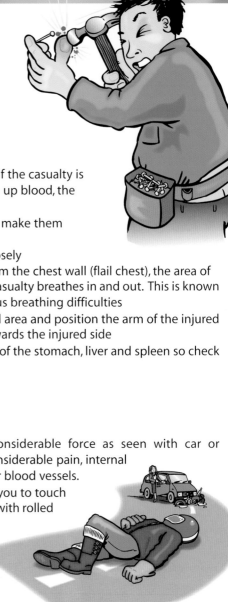

FRACTURED HANDS AND FINGERS

- Pad around the hand and fingers without applying any pressure
- Elevate the injury to reduce swelling
- Secure in place with an elevated sling
- Send to hospital or call for an ambulance

FRACTURED RIBS

This could be a fracture to a single rib or several. If the casualty is having breathing difficulties or they are coughing up blood, the ribs may have damaged the lungs.

- Place the casualty in a half-sitting position and make them comfortable
- Call 999/112 for an ambulance and monitor closely
- If the fractured ribs have become detached from the chest wall (flail chest), the area of the detached ribs will move in every time the casualty breathes in and out. This is known as paradoxical breathing and can lead to serious breathing difficulties
- In this situation, place padding over the injured area and position the arm of the injured side in an elevated sling. Lean the casualty towards the injured side
- Fractures of the lower ribs can lead to damage of the stomach, liver and spleen so check for signs of internal bleeding
- Keep the casualty warm and reassure them

FRACTURES OF THE UPPER LEG

Fractures of the thighbone (femur) require considerable force as seen with car or motorcycle accidents. This fracture will cause considerable pain, internal bleeding, and damage to muscle tissue and major blood vessels.

- It is highly unlikely that the casualty will allow you to touch the leg but if possible immobilize and support with rolled blankets or clothing
- Monitor for signs of shock
- Treat for shock but do not raise the legs
- Calm, reassure and keep the casualty warm
- Call 999/112 for an ambulance

FRACTURES OF THE LOWER LEG AND ANKLES

As there is very little skin and tissue surrounding the bones of the lower leg these fractures are often open.

- Lay the casualty down
- Treat any open wounds and bleeding, ensuring that you wear gloves
- Immobilize and support the leg in the position found with padding either side of the leg
- Call 999/112 for an ambulance
- Calm, reassure and keep warm
- Check that circulation is present beyond the injury

FRACTURES OF THE PELVIS

Injuries to the pelvis are often complicated as the pelvis provides protection for the bladder and urinary passages. Damage to these organs will cause internal bleeding that may be severe. This will undoubtedly lead to shock.

Additional signs and symptoms are:
- Pain and discomfort in the lower back and hips
- Evidence of bleeding in the urinary passage
- Difficulty in urinating

Treatment:
- Lay the casualty down and assist them to slightly bend their knees.
- Place padding underneath the knees for support
- Place padding between and around the outside of the legs to support and immobilize
- Make the casualty comfortable by placing padding under the arch of the back or any hollow of the body
- Call 999/112 for an ambulance, monitor and keep them warm
- If the casualty has to be moved to safety or an ambulance is not readily available, support the legs by tying broad-fold bandages at the knees and ankles with padding between the joints

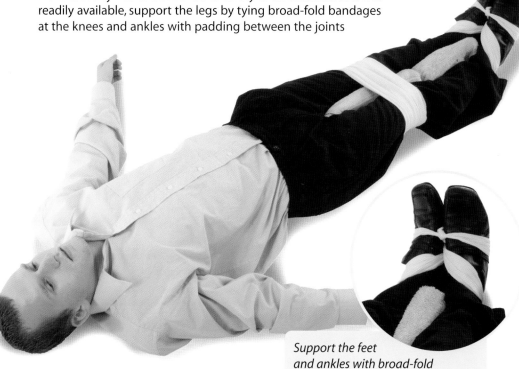

Support the feet and ankles with broad-fold bandages

FRACTURES TO THE FOOT

○ Be aware that there may be injuries to the legs if the foot is fractured
○ Lay the casualty down and raise the injured foot to reduce swelling
○ Apply a cold compress or ice pack to further reduce any swelling
○ **Do not** leave this in place for more than 10 minutes
○ **Do not** apply ice directly on the skin as this will cause a cold burn
○ **Do not** let the casualty stand or walk
○ Call for an ambulance and monitor

SPINAL INJURIES

Your spinal or vertebral column is a series of moveable bones that begin at the base of the skull and end in the centre of the hips. The spine is composed of 24 individual vertebrae, 5 sacral vertebrae which are fused to become the sacrum and 4 coccygeal vertebrae which are fused to become the coccyx. This functions as one dynamic organ upon which our structure is dependant for support and movement. Located between these vertebrae are discs that help to cushion any shock, reduce friction and allow movement. The discs do not have a direct blood supply. They receive their nutrients by osmosis and diffusion from the vertebrae. The spinal column protects the spinal cord that may become damaged if the vertebrae are fractured, dislocated or compressed.

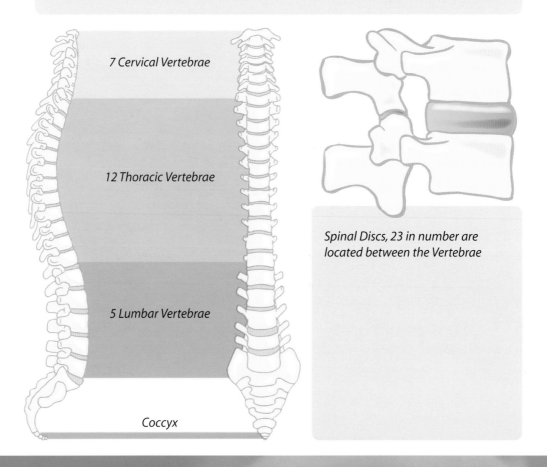

7 Cervical Vertebrae

12 Thoracic Vertebrae

5 Lumbar Vertebrae

Coccyx

Spinal Discs, 23 in number are located between the Vertebrae

WHAT CAN CAUSE A SPINAL INJURY?

- Incorrect posture and movement during manual handling of objects and people
- Slips, trips and falls
- Uneven stress on the body
- Overexertion
- Excessive weight carried
- Body posture

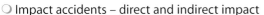

These types of injuries may cause an inability of the spine to move as a dynamic organ, leading to minor displacements of the vertebrae and discs and an irritation of the spinal nerve roots.

- Impact accidents – direct and indirect impact
- Diving accidents – swimming pools
- Collision accidents – road traffic accidents
- Sudden violent movement (rugby scrum collapsing)

These types of injuries may lead to a more permanent serious injury of the structure and the spinal cord.

Spinal injury may also arise from injuries to the chest and therefore any casualty with injuries above the base of the sternum should be treated as a spinal injury case.

TYPES OF SPINAL INJURY

VERTEBRAL FRACTURE
This could lead to a bone fragment pushing into the spinal cord.

VERTEBRAL DISLOCATION
The ligaments keeping the vertebrae in place are stretched and weakened. This will enable the vertebra to move and compress the spinal cord.

VERTEBRAL COMPRESSION
Impact injuries such as diving into a swimming pool and the head striking the pool floor could compress the vertebrae and rupture the discs.

VERTEBRAL FLEXION AND HYPEREXTENSION
This is common in whiplash injuries.

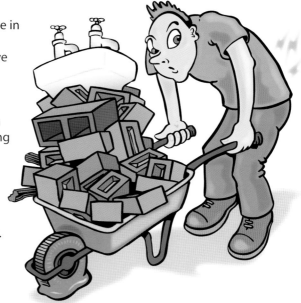

RECOGNITION OF SPINAL INJURIES

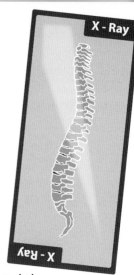

IF THE SPINAL COLUMN IS DAMAGED:
- Pain in the neck or back at the level of injury
- A step or twist in the normal curve of the spine
- Tenderness on gently feeling the spine

IF THE SPINAL CORD HAS ALSO BEEN DAMAGED:
- Loss of control of one or more limbs
- Abnormal sensations – burning or tingling
- Disorientation, anxiety, confusion
- Incontinence
- Difficulty in breathing
- The casualty may become cold and rigid

Always suspect a spinal injury if abnormal forces have been exerted on the spine i.e. violent forward or backward, bending or twisting.

Looking at the way the injury has occurred can help to predict the type and severity of injury. In many cases only those who deal with the casualty first can obtain this information – often the First Aider.

TREATMENT OF SPINAL INJURIES

THE MAIN AIMS WHEN TREATING A SUSPECTED SPINAL INJURY ARE:
- Prevent any movement
- Maintain an open airway
- Call 999/112 for an ambulance

Many casualties who have sustained partial spinal injuries are often standing and mobile, only believing that they have injured a muscle or ligament in their back or neck. Unless the casualty is immobilized the injuries could deteriorate. Movement of a casualty with spinal injuries is a last resort so leave them stabilized in the position found unless:

- You are on your own with an unconscious casualty and have to leave them to call an ambulance
- The casualty's airway is obstructed or they are vomiting
- You are unable to maintain the airway and breathing

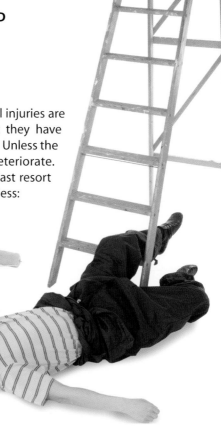

MOVING AND TURNING THE CASUALTY

The first priority here is to stabilize the head and neck in the neutral position.

From the back of the head, place your hands firmly on each side of the casualty's head with your fingers pointing towards their shoulders and positioned around the base of the skull on to the upper part of the neck.

You should be aiming to stop any movement of the head and neck.
- If you are alone, use the standard recovery position technique and try to maintain head and neck alignment
- They may have injuries, but you cannot allow the casualty's airway to be compromised
- If you have help, one person should stabilize the head and neck while the other person turns the casualty
- If there are 3 people, one person should stabilize the head and neck. The second person should turn the casualty and the third person should help to keep the back in alignment with head
- If there are 4 or more people use the log roll technique

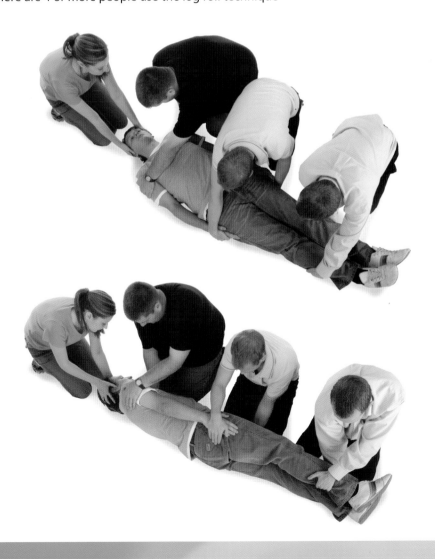

MAINTAINING THE CASUALTY'S AIRWAY

First Aiders should maintain and open the airway using a head-tilt-chin-lift manoeuvre. The jaw thrust technique is no longer recommended for First Aiders.

Protect the casualty from heat loss. Reassure them and constantly monitor for any changes in consciousness, breathing and circulation.

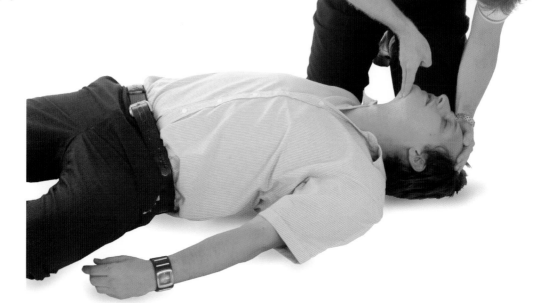

DISLOCATIONS

A strong force, an unnatural movement, or a muscle contraction can cause dislocation.

Any movement of the injured joint could also result in injury to ligaments, blood vessels and nerves.

RECOGNITION
○ Pain
○ Swelling
○ Deformity
○ Inability to move the affected area

TREATMENT
○ Treat as a fracture by supporting and immobilizing in the position found
○ Do not attempt to put the joint back in place
○ Transfer to hospital
○ Treat for shock if necessary

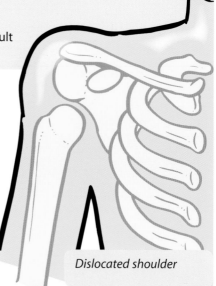

Dislocated shoulder

SOFT TISSUE INJURIES

Injuries to muscles, ligaments and tendons are often sport or activity related.

SPRAIN
This is an injury to the ligaments surrounding a joint, possibly caused by overstretching or a sudden twisting movement.

RECOGNITION
○ Pain
○ Swelling
○ Bruising
○ Inflammation of the surrounding area

STRAIN
This is a tearing injury to the muscles and tendons possibly caused by overstretching or too heavy a workload placed upon the muscles and tendons.

RECOGNITION
○ Pain
○ Swelling
○ Cramp
○ Inflammation of the surrounding area
○ Bruising

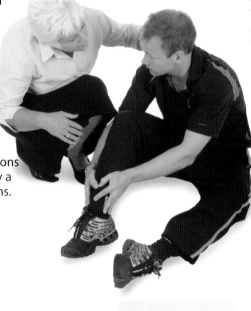

TREATMENT
Your main aims here are to reduce the pain and swelling. This will enable the casualty to make a quicker recovery.

R	REST
I	ICE
C	COMPRESS
E	ELEVATE

REST	the injured part
ICE	apply a cold compress to the injured part for approximately 10 minutes at a time
COMPRESS	the injured part firmly to reduce swelling
ELEVATE	the injured part to reduce swelling

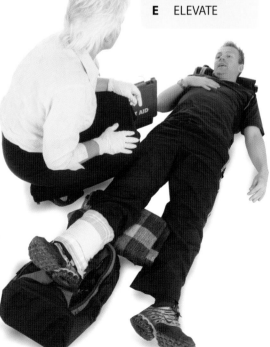

Apply ice to the injured area to reduce the swelling.

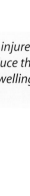

ELEVATED SLING

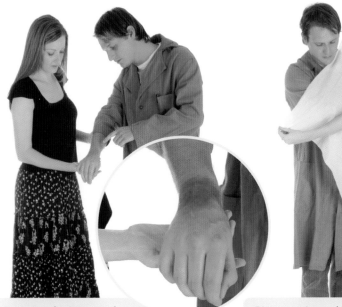

Examine the injury, ask the casualty to support the injured arm and raise the finger tips to his/her opposite shoulder.

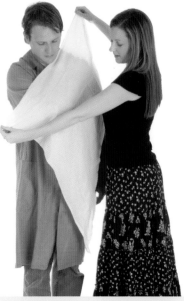

PLace a triangular bandage over the injury, with one end over the uninjured shoulder.

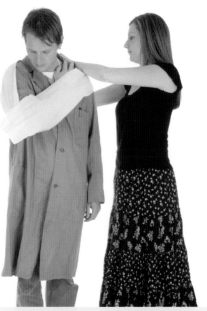

Tuck the base of the triangular bandage under the hand, forearm and elbow. Remember to leave thumb exposed so you can check circulation.

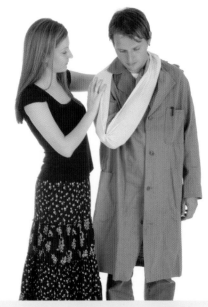

Secure at the shoulder with a reef knot. Secure at elbow with either a safety pin or twist the fabric and tuck in.

SECTION SUMMARY

WHAT CAN CAUSE A FRACTURE?
○ A direct or indirect force

WHAT ARE THE THREE MAIN TYPES OF FRACTURE?
○ Closed
○ Open
○ Complicated

WHAT IS THE BASIC TREATMENT FOR ANY FRACTURE?
○ Support and immobilize in the position found

WHAT IS A DISLOCATION?
○ When the two halves of a joint become separated

WHAT IS THE BASIC TREATMENT FOR A DISLOCATION?
○ Support and immobilise in the position found

WHAT IS THE TREATMENT FOR SOFT TISSUE INJURIES?
○ Rest
○ Ice
○ Compression
○ Elevation

IF THE SPINAL CORD BECOMES DAMAGED IN THE NECK:
○ The casualty may have respiratory and circulatory failure

HOW SHOULD YOU OPEN THE AIRWAY OF A CASUALTY WITH SUSPECTED SPINAL INJURIES?
○ Head-tilt-chin-lift maneouvre

HOW SHOULD YOU TURN A CASUALTY WITH SUSPECTED SPINAL INJURIES WHO STARTS TO VOMIT?
○ The log roll method

WHAT IS THE MINIMUM NUMBER OF PEOPLE REQUIRED TO PERFORM A LOG ROLL?
○ Four – one at the head and 3 along the body

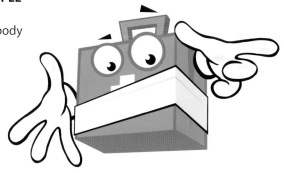

POISONING

A poison is defined as any substance entering the body in sufficient quantities that can cause temporary or permanent damage. We mostly associate poisoning with the intake of a chemical or drug that may cause direct damage to the internal organs or bodily functions. In some cases poisoning is due to substances like food or drink that we take into our bodies on a daily basis. If the quantity is too great as with alcohol poisoning, we reject the presence of a substance in our systems. The body is either unable to cope with the demand placed upon it or we produce chemicals to react against the substance and in doing so, create further complications.

HOW CAN A POISON ENTER OUR BODIES?
- By ingestion   food, drink, medicines, drugs or corrosive chemicals
- By inhalation   toxic fumes and smoke
- By injection   bites and stings, needle stick injuries or drug abuse
- By absorption chemicals and toxic vapours
- By instillation harmful substances splashed into the eyes

The recognition of poisoning is indicative of the substance entering the body and would require an entire book on the subject to explain in detail. In this chapter we will look at the recognition and treatment of poisons in the following categories:

- Household poisons
- Corrosive poisons
- Food poisoning
- Plant poisoning
- Drug poisoning
- Alcohol poisoning

FOR ALL TYPES AND ROUTES OF POISONING THE FOLLOWING RULES OF TREATMENT SHOULD BE APPLIED:
- Limit further intake of the poison
- Maintain the airway
- Identify the poison taken
- Call the emergency services

POISONING BY HOUSEHOLD CHEMICALS

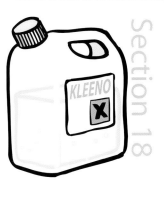

Bleach, oven cleaners, paint stripper, toilet cleaners will cause:
- Redness, blistering and burns to the skin with swelling to the face, mouth and lips if swallowed
- Distressed breathing
- Dizziness and unconsciousness

TREATMENT
- Check the airway and breathing and be prepared to carry out your procedure for Basic Life Support.
- Use a face shield when giving rescue breaths
- Identify the poison taken
- Keep them sat up and give sips of water to dilute the poison
- Certain chemicals react with water when mixed. Always have an understanding of any chemical being used in your workplace
- Do not induce vomiting
- Keep the casualty still and call 999/112 for an ambulance
- Place the unconscious casualty in the recovery position and monitor breathing

POISONING BY INDUSTRIAL CHEMICALS

Absorption, ingestion and inhalation of corrosive chemicals and gases will cause:
- Chemical burns to the skin
- Contamination of clothing and the surrounding area
- Burnt and swollen airway
- Distressed breathing
- Dizziness and unconsciousness
- Possible seizures

TREATMENT
- Remove the casualty from danger and into the fresh air if possible
- Do not put yourself in danger by entering smoke filled or contaminated areas
- Check airway and breathing and be prepared to carry out your procedure for Basic Life Support. Call 999/112 for an ambulance
- Use a face shield when giving rescue breaths
- Treat as for chemical burns
- Identify the chemical
- Place in the recovery position if unconscious and monitor breathing

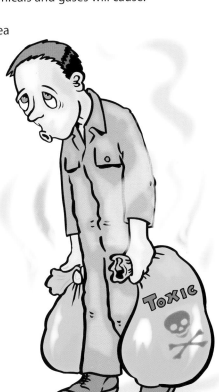

DRUG POISONING OR OVERDOSE

ASPIRIN
- Abdominal pain
- Nausea
- Vomiting (may contain blood)
- Ringing in the ears
- Confusion

PARACETAMOL
- Little effect at first
- Abdominal pain and tenderness
- Nausea
- Vomiting
- Overdose will damage the liver

ANTIDEPRESSANTS
- Shallow breathing
- Irregular pulse
- Sleepy
- Lethargy leading to unconsciousness

NARCOTICS
- Slow, shallow breathing
- Slow pulse
- Constricted pupils
- Needle marks or syringes
- Lethargy leading to unconsciousness

SOLVENTS
- Nausea
- Vomiting
- Headache
- Hallucinations
- Unconsciousness

STIMULANTS
- Sweating
- Muscle tremors
- Hallucinations
- Rapid pulse and breathing
- Strange excitable behaviour
- Rapid speech

TREATMENT
- Check airway and breathing. Be prepared to carry out your procedures for Basic Life Support. Call 999/112 for an ambulance
- Use a face shield if rescue breaths are required
- For all cases place in the recovery position
- Do not induce vomiting
- Try to obtain a sample of the drug or collect some vomit material
- Look for suicide notes
- Be aware of personality changes and violence

PLANT POISONING

There are many plants that are poisonous if swallowed or absorbed. Some are found for sale in many shops such as laburnum, iris, mistletoe and holly.
- Nausea
- Vomiting
- Headaches
- Fever and sweating

TREATMENT
As for the basic treatment of drug poisoning.

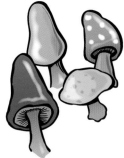

FOOD POISONING

The Salmonella or Staphylococcus groups of bacteria usually cause food poisoning. This may develop rapidly or up to 24 hours after contact with contaminated food or water.

RECOGNITION
- Nausea and vomiting
- Abdominal cramps
- Headache
- Diarrhoea
- Sweating
- Shock

TREATMENT
- Rest the casualty
- Give sips of water to re-hydrate
- Seek medical advice
- Identify the source of contamination

ALCOHOL POISONING

Alcohol, like certain drugs, can lead to depressed activity of the central nervous system with damage to the liver and kidneys if intake is prolonged.

RECOGNITION
- Nausea and vomiting
- Slow deep breathing
- Rapid pulse
- Flushed face
- Smell of alcohol
- Dry bloated face and dilated pupils
- Hypothermia
- The casualty may have sustained other injuries

TREATMENT
- Check response levels
- Check airway and breathing. Be prepared to carry out your procedures for Basic Life Support. Call 999/112 for an ambulance
- If unconscious and breathing place in the recovery position and monitor
- Keep warm and insulated from the ground
- Check for possible head injuries

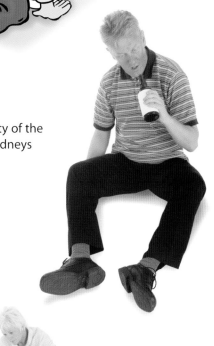

SECTION SUMMARY

WHAT IS A POISON?
○ Any substance taken in sufficient quantities that enters the body causing temporary or permanent damage

HOW CAN A POISON ENTER THE BODY?
○ Ingestion
○ Absorption
○ Injection
○ Inhalation
○ Instillation

WHAT IS THE BASIC TREATMENT FOR THE INGESTION OF A CORROSIVE POISON?
○ Keep the casualty calm and still
○ Give them sips of water or milk if there are no contra-indications
○ Call for an ambulance

WHY SHOULD YOU COLLECT A SAMPLE OF ANY POISON?
○ So that the hospital can identify the specific poison in case an antidote is required

WHAT IS THE BASIC TREATMENT FOR DRUG OR ALCOHOL POISONING?
○ Check for any danger to yourself
○ Place the casualty in the recovery position
○ Keep the casualty warm
○ Call for an ambulance
○ Be prepared to resuscitate

EFFECTS OF HEAT AND COLD

The body's thermostat that is located in the brain enables the body temperature to be monitored and to some extent controlled at a level of approximately 36.9 degrees. This does vary with the individual.

This temperature control can be affected by extremes of external heat or cold, dehydration of the body's fluid content or by injury to the head or spine that in turn affects the central nervous system.

HOW DOES THE BODY MAINTAIN ITS NORMAL TEMPERATURE?
○ The body gains heat from the conversion of food into energy (metabolism), from external heat sources and by muscle activity
○ In hot conditions blood vessels dilate allowing excess heat to be lost through the skin (sweating) and by increasing our breathing rate
○ In cold conditions the blood vessels contract which reduces sweating

THE EFFECTS OF COLD
The body reacts to cold by shutting down the blood vessels in the skin. This stops the internal or core heat from escaping.

During prolonged exposure to cold, wet and windy conditions the core body temperature may fall below 35 degrees causing normal bodily functions to slow down and eventually stop. This is known as hypothermia.

Apart from the environmental conditions, the casualty's age and general condition play a large part in the development of hypothermia, as will medical conditions such as shock and heart attack or injury to the head and spine. When treating a casualty for drowning, you should also treat for hypothermia as the body temperature falls rapidly in cold water.

RECOGNITION OF HYPOTHERMIA
○ Shivering at first that will cease as the condition progresses. This usually occurs when the body temperature is between 29 and 34 degrees
○ Cold, pale and dry skin
○ Slow shallow breathing
○ Slow weak pulse
○ Strange irrational behaviour
○ Lethargy
○ Unconsciousness leading to coma and cardiac arrest

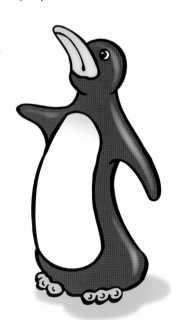

TREATMENT OF COLD CASUALTIES

Before treating for hypothermia, establish if possible, how long the casualty has been exposed to cold water or weather conditions. The length of exposure and the lower the body temperature determines the rate at which you should rewarm the casualty.

If a young healthy person falls into cold water, but is recovered quickly, they will be a cold casualty but not hypothermic. These casualties can be warmed rapidly. Remember a drop in core body temperature causes hypothermia.

Rewarming a casualty too quickly can be fatal especially if they are in poor health, have been injured or they have suffered prolonged exposure. This will result in cold blood being circulated through cold body tissue and will cause the blood to become even colder and lower blood pressure. Shock will occur and possible cardiac arrest.

Therefore, if you are treating a conscious cold casualty rewarm them by changing cold wet clothing for dry warm clothing. Give them a warm drink and assist the rewarming with blankets or extra clothes.

Do not let them move around, as this will circulate cold blood.

TREATMENT OF HYPOTHERMIA
- Remove the casualty to a sheltered and warm place
- Keep the casualty in a horizontal position
- Insulate them from the ground and surroundings
- Treat as for shock
- Cover with blankets but do not overheat
- Prevent heat escaping from the head and extremities
- Call 999/112 for an ambulance and monitor their airway and breathing
- **Do not** give any food or drink
- **Do not** rub the skin or put the casualty next to a heat source
- **Do not** stand them up or walk them around to get warm
- **Do not** overheat, warm them slowly

THE EFFECTS OF HEAT - HEAT EXHAUSTION

When the body temperature exceeds the atmospheric temperature, particularly in humid conditions, sweat will not evaporate from the body. This often takes place with strenuous exercise causing a loss of salt and water from the body (dehydration). This is known as **heat exhaustion** and because the fluid component of the blood is reduced, the casualty will suffer from shock.

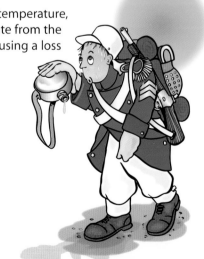

RECOGNITION
- Headache
- Confusion
- Sweating with pale, clammy skin
- Muscle cramps in the abdomen and limbs
- Rapid weakening pulse and breathing
- Temperature around 39 degrees

TREATMENT
- Place in the shade or a cool environment
- Remove outer and any restricting clothing
- Give plenty of water – 1 teaspoon of salt to a litre of water
- Lay them down and elevate the legs
- Upon recovery send to a doctor
- If the condition deteriorates call 999/112 for an ambulance
- Monitor their condition and place in the recovery position if they are unconscious and breathing

THE EFFECTS OF HEAT - HEATSTROKE
When there is a failure of the thermostat in the brain, the body's temperature will rise above 40 degrees. This may have been brought on by uncontrollable heat exhaustion, prolonged exposure to high temperatures or as a result of an illness or fever. If this is not treated immediately brain damage can occur. This is known as **heatstroke**.

RECOGNITION
- Headache
- Confusion and general discomfort
- Hot, flushed and dry skin
- Body temperature above 40 degrees (the brain starts to swell)
- Rapid deterioration
- A full, bounding pulse
- Slow and noisy breathing
- Response levels deteriorate rapidly

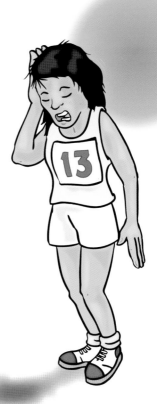

TREATMENT
- Place in the shade or a cool environment
- Remove outer clothing and cover in a cold wet sheet
- Dial 999/112 for an ambulance
- Ensure adequate ventilation or fan the casualty
- Be prepared to carry out your procedures for Basic Life Support

Heatstroke is a serious condition that can deteriorate rapidly so urgent medical attention is required.

SECTION SUMMARY

WHAT IS HYPOTHERMIA?
○ A lowering of the body's core temperature

HOW SHOULD YOU TREAT A CASUALTY WITH HYPOTHERMIA?
○ Remove the casualty to a warm place
○ Treat as for shock
○ Do not allow the casualty to stand or move around
○ Slowly raise their temperature with blankets or clothing
○ Call for an ambulance

WHY SHOULD YOU GIVE A CASUALTY SUFFERING WITH HEAT EXHAUSTION SIPS OF WATER?
○ To raise the body's fluid levels as they are dehydrated

WHAT IS HEATSTROKE?
○ A rapid, uncontrollable increase in the body's temperature caused by overexposure to heat or as a result of infection

HOW SHOULD YOU TREAT A CASUALTY WITH HEATSTROKE?
○ Lay the casualty down in a cool place and raise the head and shoulders
○ Remove outer clothing and cool the casualty by sponging them down with cold water or placing a cool wet sheet over them
○ Call for an ambulance
○ Monitor any changes in their condition

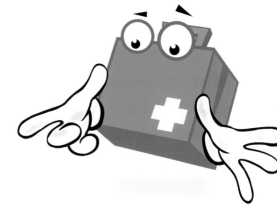

CHILD AND BABY BASIC LIFE SUPPORT

The general principles involved in the treatment of unconscious, breathing or non-breathing children and babies will be the same as with an adult but there are differences in respect of protocols. Apart from the obvious size difference, babies or infants are defined as being less than 1 year old. A child is defined as being older than 1 year of age, up to the onset of puberty. This can be difficult to establish in some cases.

If you believe the casualty to be a child, then you must adopt the protocols as defined for that of a child. If a misjudgement is made and the casualty turns out to be a young adult, little harm will come to your casualty.

As with an adult, there are numerous reasons why a baby or child may become unconscious. Generally the causes are asphyxia, either from choking or suffocation, high fever from childhood infections, diseases or convulsions.
The airway of a baby and child is smaller and shaped differently than that of an adult. Obstructions and breathing difficulties are more common.

Although children and babies can unfortunately suffer from heart conditions, the cessation of breathing or cardiac arrest is commonly due to oxygen starvation from one of the reasons noted above.

CHILD RESUSCITATION

Having assessed the surrounding areas for any danger and ensured that it is safe to approach the casualty, you should carry out a Primary Survey to identify any life threatening conditions.
- Approach the child calmly from their feet end
- Talk to them as you approach
- Kneel down by their side
- Gently tap the child's shoulders
- Speak into both ears and give a command e.g. open your eyes, talk to me
- Speak loudly and calmly

If the child is responsive but has suffered severe injuries, leave them in the position found and treat accordingly. Otherwise establish the possible cause of the collapse, treat any injuries and obtain medical assistance.

If the child does not respond shout for help to attract the attention of others.

OPENING THE AIRWAY
If the child does not respond, their airway needs protecting. If necessary turn the unconscious child into the face-up position.
- With one hand on the child's forehead tilt back the head and lift the chin with two fingers to fully open the airway
- With the airway open and maintained look, listen and feel for any signs of normal breathing for up to 10 seconds.

If the child is unconscious but breathing normally check for and treat any injuries, then place in the recovery position. Call 999/112 for an ambulance and constantly monitor the airway and breathing. If the casualty is not breathing normally ask any helpers to call 999/112 for an ambulance.

RESCUE BREATHING
- Give 5 effective rescue breaths
- With the airway open and maintained, close the nose by pinching it together. Obtain a good seal around the child's mouth. Breathe steadily into the child until the chest rises.
- Maintain the head tilt and chin lift while you allow the chest to fall and air to escape
- If you cannot inflate the chest with each inflation check the mouth for visible obstructions (NO finger sweep). Recheck the position of the head tilt and chin lift.

After giving 5 attempted, rescue breaths start CPR.

Start CPR with 30 compressions to 2 breaths. Do this for 1 minute and if no help has arrived call for an ambulance.

Locate the point on the chest as you would for the adult. Compress at a rate of 100 compressions per minute and at a depth of one third of the chest depth.

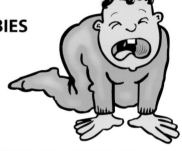

CPR ASSESSMENT CHILDREN AND BABIES

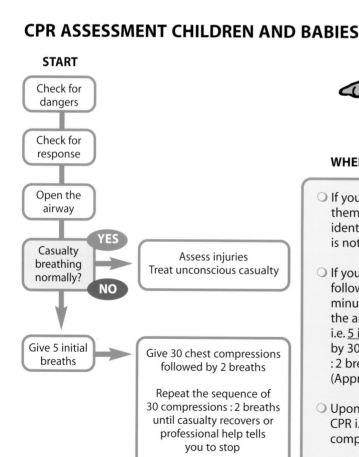

START

Check for dangers

Check for response

Open the airway

Casualty breathing normally? — **YES** → Assess injuries / Treat unconscious casualty

NO

Give 5 initial breaths → Give 30 chest compressions followed by 2 breaths

Repeat the sequence of 30 compressions : 2 breaths until casualty recovers or professional help tells you to stop

WHEN TO SUMMON HELP

- If you have help, send them as soon as you have identified that the casualty is not breathing normally

- If you have no help then follow this protocol for one minute before summoning the ambulance i.e. 5 initial breaths followed by 30 chest compressions : 2 breaths (Approx 3 cycles of 30:2)

- Upon return continue with CPR i.e. 30 chest compressions : 2 breaths

BABY RESUSCITATION

The procedures for baby resuscitation are the same as for a child but with a few variations.
- You may have to deal with distraught parents
- When checking for a response do not tap or shake the baby. Tap the hand or the sole of the foot
- Do not over extend the head and neck to obtain an open airway as you would with the child or adult. Find a neutral position
- Place one hand on the forehead and one finger under the point of the chin. Gently tilt the head back so that the mouth falls open
- Do not push into the soft flesh under the chin as this will block the airway
- Check for breathing as you would for the child but be aware that babies breathe at a faster rate

IF THE BABY IS UNCONSCIOUS BUT BREATHING NORMALLY:
You will not be able to place a baby in the standard recovery position. Hold the baby in your arms with the head tilted downwards. This will allow for any fluids to drain and the tongue to fall forwards.

IF THE BABY IS NOT BREATHING NORMALLY:
Maintain an open airway and place your lips around the baby's mouth and nose. Give 5 initial breaths. Form a good seal and breathe steadily into the baby until the chest just rises. Do this at a rate of 20 breaths per minute and do not over inflate.

Commence CPR by placing two fingers just below the line of the baby's nipples. Compress the chest with 30 compressions followed by 2 breaths. This should be done at a rate of 100 compressions per minute at a depth of a third of the chest depth. Do not over inflate the baby or press on the lower part of the breastbone.

CHOKING CHILD
As explained earlier, children and babies are prone to airway obstruction and choking. This is often caused by the presence of food, small objects or toys being lodged at the back of the mouth or in the airway.

Although the treatment here is similar to the adult, care should be taken when giving abdominal thrusts on a choking child.

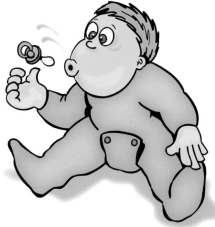

ACTION FOR A CHOKING CHILD

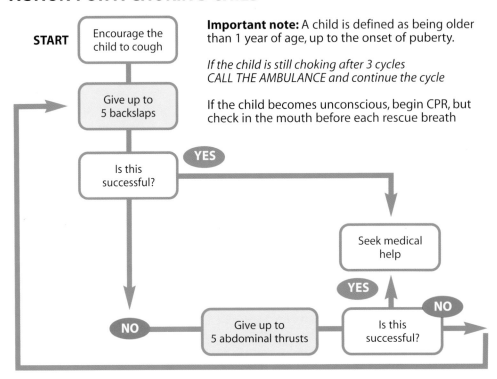

Important note: A child is defined as being older than 1 year of age, up to the onset of puberty.

*If the child is still choking after 3 cycles
CALL THE AMBULANCE and continue the cycle*

If the child becomes unconscious, begin CPR, but check in the mouth before each rescue breath

START → Encourage the child to cough → Give up to 5 backslaps → Is this successful? — YES → Seek medical help; NO → Give up to 5 abdominal thrusts → Is this successful? — YES → Seek medical help; NO →

ACTION FOR A CHOKING BABY

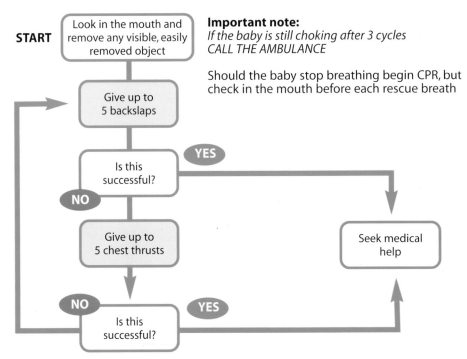

Important note:
*If the baby is still choking after 3 cycles
CALL THE AMBULANCE*

Should the baby stop breathing begin CPR, but check in the mouth before each rescue breath

START → Look in the mouth and remove any visible, easily removed object → Give up to 5 backslaps → Is this successful? — YES → Seek medical help; NO → Give up to 5 chest thrusts → Is this successful? — YES → Seek medical help; NO →

NOTES AND OBSERVATIONS

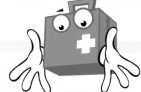

FIRST AID at work

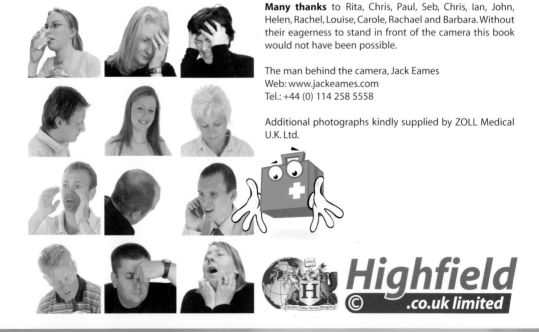

Many thanks to Rita, Chris, Paul, Seb, Chris, Ian, John, Helen, Rachel, Louise, Carole, Rachael and Barbara. Without their eagerness to stand in front of the camera this book would not have been possible.

The man behind the camera, Jack Eames
Web: www.jackeames.com
Tel.: +44 (0) 114 258 5558

Additional photographs kindly supplied by ZOLL Medical U.K. Ltd.